ACCESS YOUR ONLINE RESOURCES

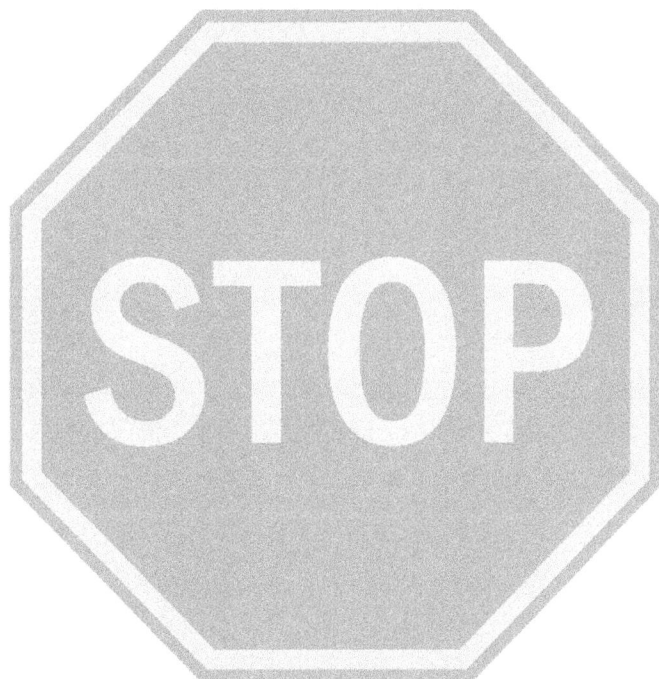

DON'T MISS OUT ON THE ONLINE RESOURCES INCLUDED WITH YOUR PURCHASE!

Your purchase of this product unlocks access to our Online Resources page. Elevate your study experience with our **interactive practice test interface**, along with all of the additional resources that we couldn't include in this book.

Flip to the Online Resources section at the end of this book to find the link and a QR code to get started!

Mometrix
TEST PREPARATION

OHST®
Exam
Secrets

Study Guide
Your Key to Exam Success

Mømetrix
TEST PREPARATION

Written and edited by the Mometrix Safety Certification Test Team

Mometrix offers volume discount pricing to institutions. For more information or a price quote, please contact our sales department at sales@mometrix.com or 888-248-1219.

OHST is a registered trademark of Board of Certified Safety Professionals, Inc., which is not affiliated with Mometrix Test Preparation and does not endorse this product.

Paperback
ISBN 13: 978-1-61072-393-0
ISBN 10: 1-61072-393-7

Ebook
ISBN 13: 978-1-62120-629-3
ISBN 10: 1-62120-629-7

Hardback
ISBN 13: 978-1-5167-1154-3
ISBN 10: 1-5167-1154-8

DEAR FUTURE EXAM SUCCESS STORY

First of all, **THANK YOU** for purchasing Mometrix study materials!

Second, congratulations! You are one of the few determined test-takers who are committed to doing whatever it takes to excel on your exam. **You have come to the right place.** We developed these study materials with one goal in mind: to deliver you the information you need in a format that's concise and easy to use.

In addition to optimizing your guide for the content of the test, we've outlined our recommended steps for breaking down the preparation process into small, attainable goals so you can make sure you stay on track.

We've also analyzed the entire test-taking process, identifying the most common pitfalls and showing how you can overcome them and be ready for any curveball the test throws you.

Standardized testing is one of the biggest obstacles on your road to success, which only increases the importance of doing well in the high-pressure, high-stakes environment of test day. Your results on this test could have a significant impact on your future, and this guide provides the information and practical advice to help you achieve your full potential on test day.

Your success is our success

We would love to hear from you! If you would like to share the story of your exam success or if you have any questions or comments in regard to our products, please contact us at **800-673-8175** or **support@mometrix.com**.

Thanks again for your business and we wish you continued success!

Sincerely,
The Mometrix Test Preparation Team

Need more help? Check out our flashcards at:
http://MometrixFlashcards.com/OHST

TABLE OF CONTENTS

Introduction

Thank you for purchasing this resource! You have made the choice to prepare yourself for a test that could have a huge impact on your future, and this guide is designed to help you be fully ready for test day. Obviously, it's important to have a solid understanding of the test material, but you also need to be prepared for the unique environment and stressors of the test, so that you can perform to the best of your abilities.

For this purpose, the first section that appears in this guide is the **Secret Keys**. We've devoted countless hours to meticulously researching what works and what doesn't, and we've boiled down our findings to the five most impactful steps you can take to improve your performance on the test. We start at the beginning with study planning and move through the preparation process, all the way to the testing strategies that will help you get the most out of what you know when you're finally sitting in front of the test.

We recommend that you start preparing for your test as far in advance as possible. However, if you've bought this guide as a last-minute study resource and only have a few days before your test, we recommend that you skip over the first two Secret Keys since they address a long-term study plan.

If you struggle with **test anxiety**, we strongly encourage you to check out our recommendations for how you can overcome it. Test anxiety is a formidable foe, but it can be beaten, and we want to make sure you have the tools you need to defeat it.

Secret Key #1 – Plan Big, Study Small

There's a lot riding on your performance. If you want to ace this test, you're going to need to keep your skills sharp and the material fresh in your mind. You need a plan that lets you review everything you need to know while still fitting in your schedule. We'll break this strategy down into three categories.

Information Organization

Start with the information you already have: the official test outline. From this, you can make a complete list of all the concepts you need to cover before the test. Organize these concepts into groups that can be studied together, and create a list of any related vocabulary you need to learn so you can brush up on any difficult terms. You'll want to keep this vocabulary list handy once you actually start studying since you may need to add to it along the way.

Time Management

Once you have your set of study concepts, decide how to spread them out over the time you have left before the test. Break your study plan into small, clear goals so you have a manageable task for each day and know exactly what you're doing. Then just focus on one small step at a time. When you manage your time this way, you don't need to spend hours at a time studying. Studying a small block of content for a short period each day helps you retain information better and avoid stressing over how much you have left to do. You can relax knowing that you have a plan to cover everything in time. In order for this strategy to be effective though, you have to start studying early and stick to your schedule. Avoid the exhaustion and futility that comes from last-minute cramming!

Study Environment

The environment you study in has a big impact on your learning. Studying in a coffee shop, while probably more enjoyable, is not likely to be as fruitful as studying in a quiet room. It's important to keep distractions to a minimum. You're only planning to study for a short block of time, so make the most of it. Don't pause to check your phone or get up to find a snack. It's also important to **avoid multitasking**. Research has consistently shown that multitasking will make your studying dramatically less effective. Your study area should also be comfortable and well-lit so you don't have the distraction of straining your eyes or sitting on an uncomfortable chair.

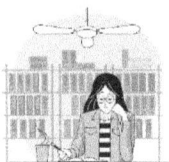

The time of day you study is also important. You want to be rested and alert. Don't wait until just before bedtime. Study when you'll be most likely to comprehend and remember. Even better, if you know what time of day your test will be, set that time aside for study. That way your brain will be used to working on that subject at that specific time and you'll have a better chance of recalling information.

Finally, it can be helpful to team up with others who are studying for the same test. Your actual studying should be done in as isolated an environment as possible, but the work of organizing the information and setting up the study plan can be divided up. In between study sessions, you can discuss with your teammates the concepts that you're all studying and quiz each other on the details. Just be sure that your teammates are as serious about the test as you are. If you find that your study time is being replaced with social time, you might need to find a new team.

Secret Key #2 – Make Your Studying Count

You're devoting a lot of time and effort to preparing for this test, so you want to be absolutely certain it will pay off. This means doing more than just reading the content and hoping you can remember it on test day. It's important to make every minute of study count. There are two main areas you can focus on to make your studying count.

Retention

It doesn't matter how much time you study if you can't remember the material. You need to make sure you are retaining the concepts. To check your retention of the information you're learning, try recalling it at later times with minimal prompting. Try carrying around flashcards and glance at one or two from time to time or ask a friend who's also studying for the test to quiz you.

To enhance your retention, look for ways to put the information into practice so that you can apply it rather than simply recalling it. If you're using the information in practical ways, it will be much easier to remember. Similarly, it helps to solidify a concept in your mind if you're not only reading it to yourself but also explaining it to someone else. Ask a friend to let you teach them about a concept you're a little shaky on (or speak aloud to an imaginary audience if necessary). As you try to summarize, define, give examples, and answer your friend's questions, you'll understand the concepts better and they will stay with you longer. Finally, step back for a big picture view and ask yourself how each piece of information fits with the whole subject. When you link the different concepts together and see them working together as a whole, it's easier to remember the individual components.

Finally, practice showing your work on any multi-step problems, even if you're just studying. Writing out each step you take to solve a problem will help solidify the process in your mind, and you'll be more likely to remember it during the test.

Modality

Modality simply refers to the means or method by which you study. Choosing a study modality that fits your own individual learning style is crucial. No two people learn best in exactly the same way, so it's important to know your strengths and use them to your advantage.

For example, if you learn best by visualization, focus on visualizing a concept in your mind and draw an image or a diagram. Try color-coding your notes, illustrating them, or creating symbols that will trigger your mind to recall a learned concept. If you learn best by hearing or discussing information, find a study partner who learns the same way or read aloud to yourself. Think about how to put the information in your own words. Imagine that you are giving a lecture on the topic and record yourself so you can listen to it later.

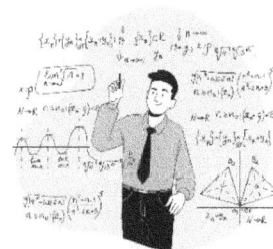

For any learning style, flashcards can be helpful. Organize the information so you can take advantage of spare moments to review. Underline key words or phrases. Use different colors for different categories. Mnemonic devices (such as creating a short list in which every item starts with the same letter) can also help with retention. Find what works best for you and use it to store the information in your mind most effectively and easily.

3

Secret Key #3 – Practice the Right Way

Your success on test day depends not only on how many hours you put into preparing, but also on whether you prepared the right way. It's good to check along the way to see if your studying is paying off. One of the most effective ways to do this is by taking practice tests to evaluate your progress. Practice tests are useful because they show exactly where you need to improve. Every time you take a practice test, pay special attention to these three groups of questions:

- The questions you got wrong
- The questions you had to guess on, even if you guessed right
- The questions you found difficult or slow to work through

This will show you exactly what your weak areas are, and where you need to devote more study time. Ask yourself why each of these questions gave you trouble. Was it because you didn't understand the material? Was it because you didn't remember the vocabulary? Do you need more repetitions on this type of question to build speed and confidence? Dig into those questions and figure out how you can strengthen your weak areas as you go back to review the material.

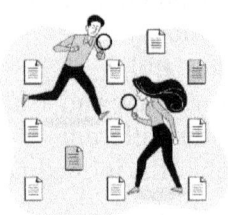

Additionally, many practice tests have a section explaining the answer choices. It can be tempting to read the explanation and think that you now have a good understanding of the concept. However, an explanation likely only covers part of the question's broader context. Even if the explanation makes perfect sense, **go back and investigate** every concept related to the question until you're positive you have a thorough understanding.

As you go along, keep in mind that the practice test is just that: practice. Memorizing these questions and answers will not be very helpful on the actual test because it is unlikely to have any of the same exact questions. If you only know the right answers to the sample questions, you won't be prepared for the real thing. **Study the concepts** until you understand them fully, and then you'll be able to answer any question that shows up on the test.

It's important to wait on the practice tests until you're ready. If you take a test on your first day of study, you may be overwhelmed by the amount of material covered and how much you need to learn. Work up to it gradually.

On test day, you'll need to be prepared for answering questions, managing your time, and using the test-taking strategies you've learned. It's a lot to balance, like a mental marathon that will have a big impact on your future. Like training for a marathon, you'll need to start slowly and work your way up. When test day arrives, you'll be ready.

Start with the strategies you've read in the first two Secret Keys—plan your course and study in the way that works best for you. If you have time, consider using multiple study resources to get different approaches to the same concepts. It can be helpful to see difficult concepts from more than one angle. Then find a good source for practice tests. Many times, the test website will suggest potential study resources or provide sample tests.

Practice Test Strategy

If you're able to find at least three practice tests, we recommend this strategy:

UNTIMED AND OPEN-BOOK PRACTICE

Take the first test with no time constraints and with your notes and study guide handy. Take your time and focus on applying the strategies you've learned.

TIMED AND OPEN-BOOK PRACTICE

Take the second practice test open-book as well, but set a timer and practice pacing yourself to finish in time.

TIMED AND CLOSED-BOOK PRACTICE

Take any other practice tests as if it were test day. Set a timer and put away your study materials. Sit at a table or desk in a quiet room, imagine yourself at the testing center, and answer questions as quickly and accurately as possible.

Keep repeating timed and closed-book tests on a regular basis until you run out of practice tests or it's time for the actual test. Your mind will be ready for the schedule and stress of test day, and you'll be able to focus on recalling the material you've learned.

Secret Key #4 – Pace Yourself

Once you're fully prepared for the material on the test, your biggest challenge on test day will be managing your time. Just knowing that the clock is ticking can make you panic even if you have plenty of time left. Work on pacing yourself so you can build confidence against the time constraints of the exam. Pacing is a difficult skill to master, especially in a high-pressure environment, so **practice is vital**.

Set time expectations for your pace based on how much time is available. For example, if a section has 60 questions and the time limit is 30 minutes, you know you have to average 30 seconds or less per question in order to answer them all. Although 30 seconds is the hard limit, set 25 seconds per question as your goal, so you reserve extra time to spend on harder questions. When you budget extra time for the harder questions, you no longer have any reason to stress when those questions take longer to answer.

Don't let this time expectation distract you from working through the test at a calm, steady pace, but keep it in mind so you don't spend too much time on any one question. Recognize that taking extra time on one question you don't understand may keep you from answering two that you do understand later in the test. If your time limit for a question is up and you're still not sure of the answer, mark it and move on, and come back to it later if the time and the test format allow. If the testing format doesn't allow you to return to earlier questions, just make an educated guess; then put it out of your mind and move on.

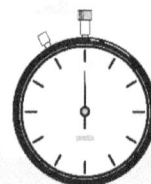

On the easier questions, be careful not to rush. It may seem wise to hurry through them so you have more time for the challenging ones, but it's not worth missing one if you know the concept and just didn't take the time to read the question fully. Work efficiently but make sure you understand the question and have looked at all of the answer choices, since more than one may seem right at first.

Even if you're paying attention to the time, you may find yourself a little behind at some point. You should speed up to get back on track, but do so wisely. Don't panic; just take a few seconds less on each question until you're caught up. Don't guess without thinking, but do look through the answer choices and eliminate any you know are wrong. If you can get down to two choices, it is often worthwhile to guess from those. Once you've chosen an answer, move on and don't dwell on any that you skipped or had to hurry through. If a question was taking too long, chances are it was one of the harder ones, so you weren't as likely to get it right anyway.

On the other hand, if you find yourself getting ahead of schedule, it may be beneficial to slow down a little. The more quickly you work, the more likely you are to make a careless mistake that will affect your score. You've budgeted time for each question, so don't be afraid to spend that time. Practice an efficient but careful pace to get the most out of the time you have.

Secret Key #5 – Have a Plan for Guessing

When you're taking the test, you may find yourself stuck on a question. Some of the answer choices seem better than others, but you don't see the one answer choice that is obviously correct. What do you do?

The scenario described above is very common, yet most test takers have not effectively prepared for it. Developing and practicing a plan for guessing may be one of the single most effective uses of your time as you get ready for the exam.

In developing your plan for guessing, there are three questions to address:

- When should you start the guessing process?
- How should you narrow down the choices?
- Which answer should you choose?

When to Start the Guessing Process

Unless your plan for guessing is to select C every time (which, despite its merits, is not what we recommend), you need to leave yourself enough time to apply your answer elimination strategies. Since you have a limited amount of time for each question, that means that if you're going to give yourself the best shot at guessing correctly, you have to decide quickly whether or not you will guess.

Of course, the best-case scenario is that you don't have to guess at all, so first, see if you can answer the question based on your knowledge of the subject and basic reasoning skills. Focus on the key words in the question and try to jog your memory of related topics. Give yourself a chance to bring the knowledge to mind, but once you realize that you don't have (or you can't access) the knowledge you need to answer the question, it's time to start the guessing process.

It's almost always better to start the guessing process too early than too late. It only takes a few seconds to remember something and answer the question from knowledge. Carefully eliminating wrong answer choices takes longer. Plus, going through the process of eliminating answer choices can actually help jog your memory.

Summary: Start the guessing process as soon as you decide that you can't answer the question based on your knowledge.

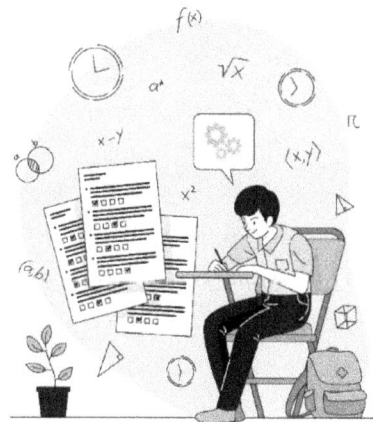

How to Narrow Down the Choices

The next chapter in this book (**Test-Taking Strategies**) includes a wide range of strategies for how to approach questions and how to look for answer choices to eliminate. You will definitely want to read those carefully, practice them, and figure out which ones work best for you. Here though, we're going to address a mindset rather than a particular strategy.

Your odds of guessing an answer correctly depend on how many options you are choosing from.

Number of options left	5	4	3	2	1
Odds of guessing correctly	20%	25%	33%	50%	100%

You can see from this chart just how valuable it is to be able to eliminate incorrect answers and make an educated guess, but there are two things that many test takers do that cause them to miss out on the benefits of guessing:

- Accidentally eliminating the correct answer
- Selecting an answer based on an impression

We'll look at the first one here, and the second one in the next section.

To avoid accidentally eliminating the correct answer, we recommend a thought exercise called **the $5 challenge**. In this challenge, you only eliminate an answer choice from contention if you are willing to bet $5 on it being wrong. Why $5? Five dollars is a small but not insignificant amount of money. It's an amount you could afford to lose but wouldn't want to throw away. And while losing $5 once might not hurt too much, doing it twenty times will set you back $100. In the same way, each small decision you make—eliminating a choice here, guessing on a question there—won't by itself impact your score very much, but when you put them all together, they can make a big difference. By holding each answer choice elimination decision to a higher standard, you can reduce the risk of accidentally eliminating the correct answer.

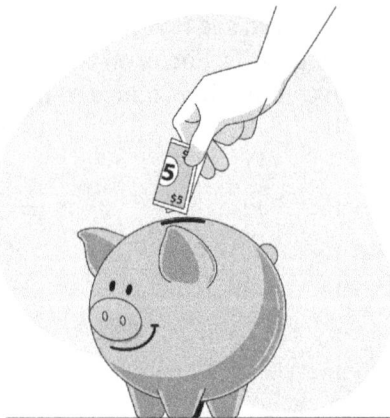

The $5 challenge can also be applied in a positive sense: If you are willing to bet $5 that an answer choice *is* correct, go ahead and mark it as correct.

Summary: Only eliminate an answer choice if you are willing to bet $5 that it is wrong.

8

Which Answer to Choose

You're taking the test. You've run into a hard question and decided you'll have to guess. You've eliminated all the answer choices you're willing to bet $5 on. Now you have to pick an answer. Why do we even need to talk about this? Why can't you just pick whichever one you feel like when the time comes?

The answer to these questions is that if you don't come into the test with a plan, you'll rely on your impression to select an answer choice, and if you do that, you risk falling into a trap. The test writers know that everyone who takes their test will be guessing on some of the questions, so they intentionally write wrong answer choices to seem plausible. You still have to pick an answer though, and if the wrong answer choices are designed to look right, how can you ever be sure that you're not falling for their trap? The best solution we've found to this dilemma is to take the decision out of your hands entirely. Here is the process we recommend:

Once you've eliminated any choices that you are confident (willing to bet $5) are wrong, select the first remaining choice as your answer.

Whether you choose to select the first remaining choice, the second, or the last, the important thing is that you use some preselected standard. Using this approach guarantees that you will not be enticed into selecting an answer choice that looks right, because you are not basing your decision on how the answer choices look.

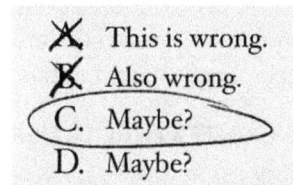

This is not meant to make you question your knowledge. Instead, it is to help you recognize the difference between your knowledge and your impressions. There's a huge difference between thinking an answer is right because of what you know, and thinking an answer is right because it looks or sounds like it should be right.

Summary: To ensure that your selection is appropriately random, make a predetermined selection from among all answer choices you have not eliminated.

Test-Taking Strategies

This section contains a list of test-taking strategies that you may find helpful as you work through the test. By taking what you know and applying logical thought, you can maximize your chances of answering any question correctly!

It is very important to realize that every question is different and every person is different: no single strategy will work on every question, and no single strategy will work for every person. That's why we've included all of them here, so you can try them out and determine which ones work best for different types of questions and which ones work best for you.

Question Strategies

⊘ READ CAREFULLY

Read the question and the answer choices carefully. Don't miss the question because you misread the terms. You have plenty of time to read each question thoroughly and make sure you understand what is being asked. Yet a happy medium must be attained, so don't waste too much time. You must read carefully and efficiently.

⊘ CONTEXTUAL CLUES

Look for contextual clues. If the question includes a word you are not familiar with, look at the immediate context for some indication of what the word might mean. Contextual clues can often give you all the information you need to decipher the meaning of an unfamiliar word. Even if you can't determine the meaning, you may be able to narrow down the possibilities enough to make a solid guess at the answer to the question.

⊘ PREFIXES

If you're having trouble with a word in the question or answer choices, try dissecting it. Take advantage of every clue that the word might include. Prefixes can be a huge help. Usually, they allow you to determine a basic meaning. *Pre-* means before, *post-* means after, *pro-* is positive, *de-* is negative. From prefixes, you can get an idea of the general meaning of the word and try to put it into context.

⊘ HEDGE WORDS

Watch out for critical hedge words, such as *likely, may, can, often, almost, mostly, usually, generally, rarely,* and *sometimes.* Question writers insert these hedge phrases to cover every possibility. Often an answer choice will be wrong simply because it leaves no room for exception. Be on guard for answer choices that have definitive words such as *exactly* and *always.*

⊘ SWITCHBACK WORDS

Stay alert for *switchbacks.* These are the words and phrases frequently used to alert you to shifts in thought. The most common switchback words are *but, although,* and *however.* Others include *nevertheless, on the other hand, even though, while, in spite of, despite,* and *regardless of.* Switchback words are important to catch because they can change the direction of the question or an answer choice.

⊘ FACE VALUE

When in doubt, use common sense. Accept the situation in the problem at face value. Don't read too much into it. These problems will not require you to make wild assumptions. If you have to go beyond creativity and warp time or space in order to have an answer choice fit the question, then you should move on and consider the other answer choices. These are normal problems rooted in reality. The applicable relationship or explanation may not be readily apparent, but it is there for you to figure out. Use your common sense to interpret anything that isn't clear.

Answer Choice Strategies

⊘ ANSWER SELECTION

The most thorough way to pick an answer choice is to identify and eliminate wrong answers until only one is left, then confirm it is the correct answer. Sometimes an answer choice may immediately seem right, but be careful. The test writers will usually put more than one reasonable answer choice on each question, so take a second to read all of them and make sure that the other choices are not equally obvious. As long as you have time left, it is better to read every answer choice than to pick the first one that looks right without checking the others.

⊘ ANSWER CHOICE FAMILIES

An answer choice family consists of two (in rare cases, three) answer choices that are very similar in construction and cannot all be true at the same time. If you see two answer choices that are direct opposites or parallels, one of them is usually the correct answer. For instance, if one answer choice says that quantity x increases and another either says that quantity x decreases (opposite) or says that quantity y increases (parallel), then those answer choices would fall into the same family. An answer choice that doesn't match the construction of the answer choice family is more likely to be incorrect. Most questions will not have answer choice families, but when they do appear, you should be prepared to recognize them.

⊘ ELIMINATE ANSWERS

Eliminate answer choices as soon as you realize they are wrong, but make sure you consider all possibilities. If you are eliminating answer choices and realize that the last one you are left with is also wrong, don't panic. Start over and consider each choice again. There may be something you missed the first time that you will realize on the second pass.

⊘ AVOID FACT TRAPS

Don't be distracted by an answer choice that is factually true but doesn't answer the question. You are looking for the choice that answers the question. Stay focused on what the question is asking for so you don't accidentally pick an answer that is true but incorrect. Always go back to the question and make sure the answer choice you've selected actually answers the question and is not merely a true statement.

⊘ EXTREME STATEMENTS

In general, you should avoid answers that put forth extreme actions as standard practice or proclaim controversial ideas as established fact. An answer choice that states the "process should be used in certain situations, if..." is much more likely to be correct than one that states the "process should be discontinued completely." The first is a calm rational statement and doesn't even make a definitive, uncompromising stance, using a hedge word *if* to provide wiggle room, whereas the second choice is far more extreme.

⊘ BENCHMARK

As you read through the answer choices and you come across one that seems to answer the question well, mentally select that answer choice. This is not your final answer, but it's the one that will help you evaluate the other answer choices. The one that you selected is your benchmark or standard for judging each of the other answer choices. Every other answer choice must be compared to your benchmark. That choice is correct until proven otherwise by another answer choice beating it. If you find a better answer, then that one becomes your new benchmark. Once you've decided that no other choice answers the question as well as your benchmark, you have your final answer.

⊘ PREDICT THE ANSWER

Before you even start looking at the answer choices, it is often best to try to predict the answer. When you come up with the answer on your own, it is easier to avoid distractions and traps because you will know exactly what to look for. The right answer choice is unlikely to be word-for-word what you came up with, but it should be a close match. Even if you are confident that you have the right answer, you should still take the time to read each option before moving on.

General Strategies

⊘ TOUGH QUESTIONS

If you are stumped on a problem or it appears too hard or too difficult, don't waste time. Move on! Remember though, if you can quickly check for obviously incorrect answer choices, your chances of guessing correctly are greatly improved. Before you completely give up, at least try to knock out a couple of possible answers. Eliminate what you can and then guess at the remaining answer choices before moving on.

⊘ CHECK YOUR WORK

Since you will probably not know every term listed and the answer to every question, it is important that you get credit for the ones that you do know. Don't miss any questions through careless mistakes. If at all possible, try to take a second to look back over your answer selection and make sure you've selected the correct answer choice and haven't made a costly careless mistake (such as marking an answer choice that you didn't mean to mark). This quick double check should more than pay for itself in caught mistakes for the time it costs.

⊘ PACE YOURSELF

It's easy to be overwhelmed when you're looking at a page full of questions; your mind is confused and full of random thoughts, and the clock is ticking down faster than you would like. Calm down and maintain the pace that you have set for yourself. Especially as you get down to the last few minutes of the test, don't let the small numbers on the clock make you panic. As long as you are on track by monitoring your pace, you are guaranteed to have time for each question.

⊘ DON'T RUSH

It is very easy to make errors when you are in a hurry. Maintaining a fast pace in answering questions is pointless if it makes you miss questions that you would have gotten right otherwise. Test writers like to include distracting information and wrong answers that seem right. Taking a little extra time to avoid careless mistakes can make all the difference in your test score. Find a pace that allows you to be confident in the answers that you select.

⊘ Keep Moving

Panicking will not help you pass the test, so do your best to stay calm and keep moving. Taking deep breaths and going through the answer elimination steps you practiced can help to break through a stress barrier and keep your pace.

Final Notes

The combination of a solid foundation of content knowledge and the confidence that comes from practicing your plan for applying that knowledge is the key to maximizing your performance on test day. As your foundation of content knowledge is built up and strengthened, you'll find that the strategies included in this chapter become more and more effective in helping you quickly sift through the distractions and traps of the test to isolate the correct answer.

Now that you're preparing to move forward into the test content chapters of this book, be sure to keep your goal in mind. As you read, think about how you will be able to apply this information on the test. If you've already seen sample questions for the test and you have an idea of the question format and style, try to come up with questions of your own that you can answer based on what you're reading. This will give you valuable practice applying your knowledge in the same ways you can expect to on test day.

Good luck and good studying!

Fundamental Math and Science and Business Calculations/Analysis

Algebra

EQUATIONS AND GRAPHING

When algebraic functions and equations are shown graphically, they are usually shown on a *Cartesian Coordinate Plane*. The Cartesian coordinate plane consists of two number lines placed perpendicular to each other, and intersecting at the zero point, also known as the origin. The horizontal number line is known as the x-axis, with positive values to the right of the origin, and negative values to the left of the origin. The vertical number line is known as the y-axis, with positive values above the origin, and negative values below the origin. Any point on the plane can be identified by an ordered pair in the form (x,y), called coordinates. The x-value of the coordinate is called the abscissa, and the y-value of the coordinate is called the ordinate. The two number lines divide the plane into four quadrants: I, II, III, and IV.

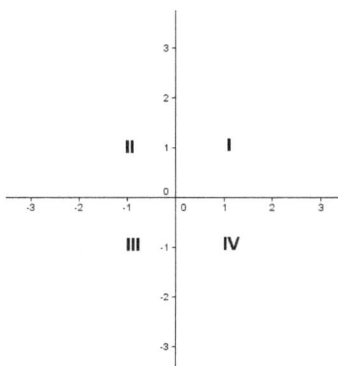

> **Review Video: <u>Cartesian Coordinate Plane and Graphing</u>**
> Visit mometrix.com/academy and enter code: 115173

Before learning the different forms equations can be written in, it is important to understand some terminology. A ratio of the change in the vertical distance to the change in horizontal distance is called the *Slope*. On a graph with two points, (x_1, y_1) and (x_2, y_2), the slope is represented by the formula $= \frac{y_2 - y_1}{x_2 - x_1}$; $x_1 \neq x_2$. If the value of the slope is positive, the line slopes upward from left to right. If the value of the slope is negative, the line slopes downward from left to right. If the y-coordinates are the same for both points, the slope is 0 and the line is a *Horizontal Line*. If the x-coordinates are the same for both points, there is no slope and the line is a *Vertical Line*. Two or more lines that have equal slopes are *Parallel Lines*. *Perpendicular Lines* have slopes that are negative reciprocals of each other, such as $\frac{a}{b}$ and $\frac{-b}{a}$.

Equations are made up of monomials and polynomials. A *Monomial* is a single constant, variable, or product of constants and variables, such as 7, x, $2x$, or x^3y. There will never be addition or subtraction symbols in a monomial. Like monomials have like variables, but they may have different coefficients. *Polynomials* are algebraic expressions which use addition and subtraction to combine two or more monomials. Two terms make a binomial; three terms make a trinomial; etc..

15

The *Degree of a Monomial* is the sum of the exponents of the variables. The *Degree of a Polynomial* is the highest degree of any individual term.

As mentioned previously, equations can be written many ways. Below is a list of the many forms equations can take.

- Standard Form: $Ax + By = C$; the slope is $\frac{-A}{B}$ and the y-intercept is $\frac{C}{B}$
- *Slope Intercept Form*: $y = mx + b$, where m is the slope and b is the y-intercept
- Point-Slope Form: $y - y_1 = m(x - x_1)$, where m is the slope and (x_1, y_1) is a point on the line
- Two-Point Form: $\frac{y-y_1}{x-x_1} = \frac{y_2-y_1}{x_2-x_1}$, where (x_1, y_1) and (x_2, y_2) are two points on the given line
- *Intercept Form*: $\frac{x}{x_1} + \frac{y}{y_1} = 1$, where $(x_1, 0)$ is the point at which a line intersects the x-axis, and $(0, y_1)$ is the point at which the same line intersects the y-axis

Equations that can be written as $ax + b = 0$, where $a \neq 0$, are referred to as **one variable linear equations**. A solution to such an equation is called a **root**. In the case where we have the equation $5x + 10 = 0$, if we solve for x we get a solution of $x = -2$. In other words, the root of the equation is -2. This is found by first subtracting 10 from both sides, which gives $5x = -10$. Next, simply divide both sides by the coefficient of the variable, in this case 5, to get $x = -2$. This can be checked by plugging -2 back into the original equation $(5)(-2) + 10 = -10 + 10 = 0$.

The **solution set** is the set of all solutions of an equation. In our example, the solution set would simply be -2. If there were more solutions (there usually are in multivariable equations) then they would also be included in the solution set. When an equation has no true solutions, it is referred to as an **empty set**. Equations with identical solution sets are **equivalent equations**. An **identity** is a term whose value or determinant is equal to 1.

> **Review Video: <u>Linear Equations Basics</u>**
> Visit mometrix.com/academy and enter code: 793005

OTHER IMPORTANT CONCEPTS

Commonly in algebra and other upper-level fields of math you find yourself working with mathematical expressions that do not equal each other. The statement comparing such expressions with symbols such as < (less than) or > (greater than) is called an *Inequality*. An example of an inequality is $7x > 5$. To solve for x, simply divide both sides by 7 and the solution is shown to be $x > \frac{5}{7}$. Graphs of the solution set of inequalities are represented on a number line. Open circles are used to show that an expression approaches a number but is never quite equal to that number.

Conditional Inequalities are those with certain values for the variable that will make the condition true and other values for the variable where the condition will be false. *Absolute Inequalities* can have any real number as the value for the variable to make the condition true, while there is no real number value for the variable that will make the condition false. Solving inequalities is done by following the same rules as for solving equations with the exception that when multiplying or dividing by a negative number the direction of the inequality sign must be flipped or reversed. *Double Inequalities* are situations where two inequality statements apply to the same variable expression. An example of this is $-c < ax + b < c$.

A *Weighted Mean*, or weighted average, is a mean that uses "weighted" values. The formula is weighted mean $= \frac{w_1 x_1 + w_2 x_2 + w_3 x_3 \ldots + w_n x_n}{w_1 + w_2 + w_3 + \cdots + w_n}$. Weighted values, such as $w_1, w_2, w_3, \ldots w_n$ are assigned to each member of the set $x_1, x_2, x_3, \ldots x_n$. When calculating the weighted mean, make sure a weight value for each member of the set is used.

> **Review Video: Conditional and Absolute Inequalities**
> Visit mometrix.com/academy and enter code: 980164

CALCULATIONS USING POINTS

Sometimes you need to perform calculations using only points on a graph as input data. Using points, you can determine what the midpoint and distance are. If you know the equation for a line you can calculate the distance between the line and the point.

To find the *Midpoint* of two points (x_1, y_1) and (x_2, y_2), average the x-coordinates to get the x-coordinate of the midpoint, and average the y-coordinates to get the y-coordinate of the midpoint. The formula is midpoint $= \left(\frac{x_1 + x_2}{2}, \frac{y_1 + y_2}{2} \right)$.

The *Distance* between two points is the same as the length of the hypotenuse of a right triangle with the two given points as endpoints, and the two sides of the right triangle parallel to the x-axis and y-axis, respectively. The length of the segment parallel to the x-axis is the difference between the x-coordinates of the two points. The length of the segment parallel to the y-axis is the difference between the y-coordinates of the two points. Use the Pythagorean Theorem $a^2 + b^2 = c^2$ or $c = \sqrt{a^2 + b^2}$ to find the distance. The formula is: distance $= \sqrt{(x_2 - x_1)^2 + (y_2 - y_1)^2}$.

When a line is in the format $Ax + By + C = 0$, where A, B, and C are coefficients, you can use a point (x_1, y_1) not on the line and apply the formula $d = \frac{|Ax_1 + By_1 + C|}{\sqrt{A^2 + B^2}}$ to find the distance between the line and the point (x_1, y_1).

> **Review Video: Calculations Using Points on a Graph**
> Visit mometrix.com/academy and enter code: 883228

SYSTEMS OF EQUATIONS

Systems of Equations are a set of simultaneous equations that all use the same variables. A solution to a system of equations must be true for each equation in the system. *Consistent Systems* are those with at least one solution. *Inconsistent Systems* are systems of equations that have no solution.

To solve a system of linear equations by **substitution**, start with the easier equation and solve for one of the variables. Express this variable in terms of the other variable. Substitute this expression in the other equation and solve for the other variable. The solution should be expressed in the form (x, y). Substitute the values into both of the original equations to check your answer. Consider the following system of equations:

$$x + 6y = 15$$
$$3x - 12y = 18$$

Solving the first equation for x: $x = 15 - 6y$

Substitute this value in place of x in the second equation, and solve for y:

$$3(15 - 6y) - 12y = 18$$
$$45 - 18y - 12y = 18$$
$$30y = 27$$
$$y = \frac{27}{30} = \frac{9}{10} = 0.9$$

Plug this value for y back into the first equation to solve for x:

$$x = 15 - 6(0.9) = 15 - 5.4 = 9.6$$

Check both equations if you have time:

$$9.6 + 6(0.9) = 15 \qquad 3(9.6) - 12(0.9) = 18$$
$$9.6 + 5.4 = 15 \qquad 28.8 - 10.8 = 18$$
$$15 = 15 \qquad 18 = 18$$

Therefore, the solution is (9.6,0.9).

> **Review Video: The Substitution Method**
> Visit mometrix.com/academy and enter code: 565151

To solve a system of equations using *elimination*, begin by rewriting both equations in standard form $Ax + By = C$. Check to see if the coefficients of one pair of like variables add to zero. If not, multiply one or both of the equations by a non-zero number to make one set of like variables add to zero. Add the two equations to solve for one of the variables. Substitute this value into one of the original equations to solve for the other variable. Check your work by substituting into the other equation. Next, we will solve the same problem as above, but using the addition method.

Solve the system using elimination:

$$x + 6y = 15$$
$$3x - 12y = 18$$

If we multiply the first equation by 2, we can eliminate the y terms:

$$2x + 12y = 30$$
$$3x - 12y = 18$$

Add the equations together and solve for x:

$$5x = 48$$

$$x = \frac{48}{5} = 9.6$$

Plug the value for x back into either of the original equations and solve for y:

$$9.6 + 6y = 15$$

$$y = \frac{15 - 9.6}{6} = 0.9$$

18

Check both equations if you have time:

$$9.6 + 6(0.9) = 9.6 + 5.4 = 15$$
$$3(9.6) - 12(0.9) = 28.8 - 10.8 = 18$$

Therefore, the solution is (9.6, 0.9).

> **Review Video: Substitution and Elimination for Solving Linear Systems**
> Visit mometrix.com/academy and enter code: 958611

POLYNOMIAL ALGEBRA

To multiply two binomials, follow the *FOIL* method. FOIL stands for:

- First: Multiply the first term of each binomial
- Outer: Multiply the outer terms of each binomial
- Inner: Multiply the inner terms of each binomial
- Last: Multiply the last term of each binomial

Using FOIL, $(Ax + By)(Cx + Dy) = ACx^2 + ADxy + BCxy + BDy^2$.

To divide polynomials, begin by arranging the terms of each polynomial in order of one variable. You may arrange in ascending or descending order, but be consistent with both polynomials. To get the first term of the quotient, divide the first term of the dividend by the first term of the divisor. Multiply the first term of the quotient by the entire divisor and subtract that product from the dividend. Repeat for the second and successive terms until you either get a remainder of zero or a remainder whose degree is less than the degree of the divisor. If the quotient has a remainder, write the answer as a mixed expression in the form: quotient $+ \frac{\text{remainder}}{\text{divisor}}$.

Rational Expressions are fractions with polynomials in both the numerator and the denominator; the value of the polynomial in the denominator cannot be equal to zero. To add or subtract rational expressions, first find the common denominator, then rewrite each fraction as an equivalent fraction with the common denominator. Finally, add or subtract the numerators to get the numerator of the answer, and keep the common denominator as the denominator of the answer. When multiplying rational expressions factor each polynomial and cancel like factors (a factor which appears in both the numerator and the denominator). Then, multiply all remaining factors in the numerator to get the numerator of the product, and multiply the remaining factors in the denominator to get the denominator of the product. Remember – cancel entire factors, not individual terms. To divide rational expressions, take the reciprocal of the divisor (the rational expression you are dividing by) and multiply by the dividend.

> **Review Video: Rational Expressions**
> Visit mometrix.com/academy and enter code: 415183

Below are patterns of some special products to remember: *perfect trinomial squares*, the *difference between two squares*, the *sum and difference of two cubes*, and *perfect cubes*.

- Perfect Trinomial Squares: $x^2 + 2xy + y^2 = (x + y)^2$ or $x^2 - 2xy + y^2 = (x - y)^2$
- Difference between Two Squares: $x^2 - y^2 = (x + y)(x - y)$
- Sum of Two Cubes: $x^3 + y^3 = (x + y)(x^2 - xy + y^2)$
  Note: the second factor is NOT the same as a perfect trinomial square, so do not try to factor it further.

- Difference between Two Cubes: $x^3 - y^3 = (x - y)(x^2 + xy + y^2)$
  Again, the second factor is NOT the same as a perfect trinomial square.
- Perfect Cubes: $x^3 + 3x^2y + 3xy^2 + y^3 = (x + y)^3$ and $x^3 - 3x^2y + 3xy^2 - y^3 = (x - y)^3$

In order to *factor* a polynomial, first check for a common monomial factor. When the greatest common monomial factor has been factored out, look for patterns of special products: differences of two squares, the sum or difference of two cubes for binomial factors, or perfect trinomial squares for trinomial factors. If the factor is a trinomial but not a perfect trinomial square, look for a factorable form, such as $x^2 + (a + b)x + ab = (x + a)(x + b)$ or $(ac)x^2 + (ad + bc)x + bd = (ax + b)(cx + d)$. For factors with four terms, look for groups to factor. Once you have found the factors, write the original polynomial as the product of all the factors. Make sure all of the polynomial factors are prime. Monomial factors may be prime or composite. Check your work by multiplying the factors to make sure you get the original polynomial.

SOLVING QUADRATIC EQUATIONS

The *Quadratic Formula* is used to solve quadratic equations when other methods are more difficult. To use the quadratic formula to solve a quadratic equation, begin by rewriting the equation in standard form $ax^2 + bx + c = 0$, where a, b, and c are coefficients. Once you have identified the values of the coefficients, substitute those values into the quadratic formula $x = \frac{-b \pm \sqrt{b^2 - 4ac}}{2a}$. Evaluate the equation and simplify the expression. Again, check each root by substituting into the original equation. In the quadratic formula, the portion of the formula under the radical ($b^2 - 4ac$) is called the *Discriminant*. If the discriminant is zero, there is only one root: zero. If the discriminant is positive, there are two different real roots. If the discriminant is negative, there are no real roots.

To solve a quadratic equation by *Factoring*, begin by rewriting the equation in standard form, if necessary. Factor the side with the variable then set each of the factors equal to zero and solve the resulting linear equations. Check your answers by substituting the roots you found into the original equation. If, when writing the equation in standard form, you have an equation in the form $x^2 + c = 0$ or $x^2 - c = 0$, set $x^2 = -c$ or $x^2 = c$ and take the square root of c. If $c = 0$, the only real root is zero. If c is positive, there are two real roots—the positive and negative square root values. If c is negative, there are no real roots because you cannot take the square root of a negative number.

To solve a quadratic equation by *Completing the Square*, rewrite the equation so that all terms containing the variable are on the left side of the equal sign, and all the constants are on the right side of the equal sign. Make sure the coefficient of the squared term is 1. If there is a coefficient with the squared term, divide each term on both sides of the equal side by that number. Next, work with the coefficient of the single-variable term. Square half of this coefficient, and add that value to both sides. Now you can factor the left side (the side containing the variable) as the square of a binomial. $x^2 + 2ax + a^2 = C \Rightarrow (x + a)^2 = C$, where x is the variable, and a and C are constants. Take the square root of both sides and solve for the variable. Substitute the value of the variable in the original problem to check your work.

RATIOS

A ratio is a comparison of two quantities in a particular order. Example: If there are 14 computers in a lab, and the class has 20 students, there is a student to computer ratio of 20 to 14, commonly written as 20:14.

Two more comparisons used frequently in algebra are ratios and proportions. A *Ratio* is a comparison of two quantities, expressed in a number of different ways. Ratios can be listed as "a to b", "a:b", or "a/b". Examples of ratios are miles per hour (miles/hour), meters per second (meters/second), miles per gallon (miles/gallon), etc.

Review Video: Ratios
Visit mometrix.com/academy and enter code: 996914

Geometry

PYTHAGOREAN THEOREM

The side of a triangle opposite the right angle is called the hypotenuse. The other two sides are called the legs. The Pythagorean Theorem states a relationship among the legs and hypotenuse of a right triangle: $a^2 + b^2 = c^2$, where a and b are the lengths of the legs of a right triangle, and c is the length of the hypotenuse. Note that this formula will only work with right triangles.

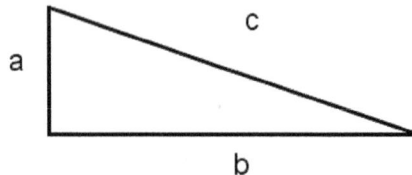

Review Video: **Pythagorean Theorem**
Visit mometrix.com/academy and enter code: 906576

AREA AND PERIMETER FORMULAS

The perimeter of any triangle is found by summing the three side lengths; $P = a + b + c$. For an equilateral triangle, this is the same as $P = 3s$, where s is any side length, since all three sides are the same length.

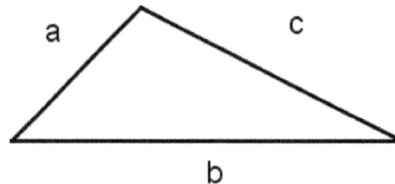

The area of any triangle can be found by taking half the product of one side length (base or b) and the perpendicular distance from that side to the opposite vertex (height or h). In equation form, $A = \frac{1}{2}bh$. For many triangles, it may be difficult to calculate h, so using one of the other formulas given here may be easier.

Another formula that works for any triangle is $A = \sqrt{s(s-a)(s-b)(s-c)}$, where A is the area, s is the semiperimeter $s = \frac{a+b+c}{2}$, and a, b, and c are the lengths of the three sides.

The area of an equilateral triangle can be found by the formula $A = \frac{\sqrt{3}}{4}s^2$, where A is the area and s is the length of a side. You could use the $30° - 60° - 90°$ ratios to find the height of the triangle and then use the standard triangle area formula, but this is faster.

The area of an isosceles triangle can be found by the formula, $A = \frac{1}{2}b\sqrt{a^2 - \frac{b^2}{4}}$, where A is the area, b is the base (the unique side), and a is the length of one of the two congruent sides. If you do not remember this formula, you can use the Pythagorean Theorem to find the height so you can use the standard formula for the area of a triangle.

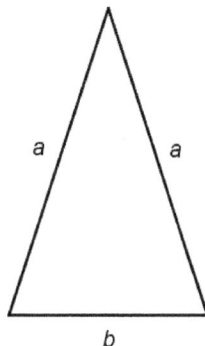

TRIGONOMETRIC FORMULAS

In the diagram below, angle C is the right angle, and side c is the hypotenuse. Side a is the side adjacent to angle B and side b is the side adjacent to angle A. These formulas will work for any acute angle in a right triangle. They will NOT work for any triangle that is not a right triangle. Also, they will not work for the right angle in a right triangle, since there are not distinct adjacent and opposite sides to differentiate from the hypotenuse.

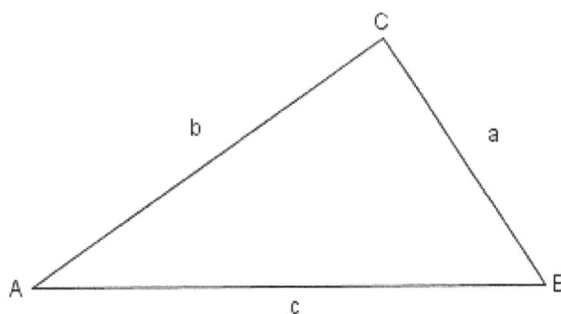

$$\sin A = \frac{\text{opposite side}}{\text{hypotenuse}} = \frac{a}{c}$$

$$\cos A = \frac{\text{adjacent side}}{\text{hypotenuse}} = \frac{b}{c}$$

$$\tan A = \frac{\text{opposite side}}{\text{adjacent side}} = \frac{a}{b}$$

$$\csc A = \frac{1}{\sin A} = \frac{\text{hypotenuse}}{\text{opposite side}} - \frac{c}{a}$$

$$\sec A = \frac{1}{\cos A} = \frac{\text{hypotenuse}}{\text{adjacent side}} = \frac{c}{b}$$

$$\cot A = \frac{1}{\tan A} = \frac{\text{adjacent side}}{\text{opposite side}} = \frac{b}{a}$$

23

LAWS OF SINES AND COSINES

The Law of Sines states that $\frac{\sin A}{a} = \frac{\sin B}{b} = \frac{\sin C}{c}$, where A, B, and C are the angles of a triangle, and a, b, and c are the sides opposite their respective angles. This formula will work with all triangles, not just right triangles.

Review Video: Law of Sines
Visit mometrix.com/academy and enter code: 206844

The Law of Cosines is given by the formula $c^2 = a^2 + b^2 - 2ab(\cos C)$, where a, b, and c are the sides of a triangle, and C is the angle opposite side c. This formula is similar to the Pythagorean Theorem, but unlike the Pythagorean Theorem, it can be used on any triangle.

CIRCLES

The center is the single point inside the circle that is equidistant from every point on the circle. (Point O in the diagram below.)

The radius is a line segment that joins the center of the circle and any one point on the circle. All radii of a circle are equal. (Segments OX, OY, and OZ in the diagram below.)

The diameter is a line segment that passes through the center of the circle and has both endpoints on the circle. The length of the diameter is exactly twice the length of the radius. (Segment XZ in the diagram below.)

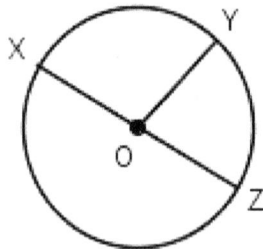

The area of a circle is found by the formula $A = \pi r^2$, where r is the length of the radius. If the diameter of the circle is given, remember to divide it in half to get the length of the radius before proceeding.

The circumference of a circle is found by the formula $C = 2\pi r$, where r is the radius. Again, remember to convert the diameter if you are given that measure rather than the radius.

Review Video: Area and Circumference of a Circle
Visit mometrix.com/academy and enter code: 243015

SOLIDS

The surface area of a solid object is the area of all sides or exterior surfaces. For objects such as prisms and pyramids, a further distinction is made between base surface area (B) and lateral surface area (LA). For a prism, the total surface area (SA) is $SA = LA + 2B$. For a pyramid or cone, the total surface area is $SA = LA + B$.

The surface area of a sphere can be found by the formula $A = 4\pi r^2$, where r is the radius. The volume is given by the formula $V = \frac{4}{3}\pi r^3$, where r is the radius. Both quantities are generally given in terms of π.

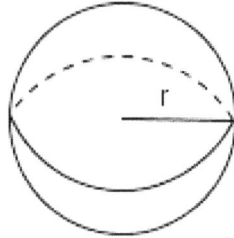

The volume of a cube can be found by the formula $V = s^3$, where s is the length of a side. The surface area of a cube is calculated as $SA = 6s^2$, where SA is the total surface area and s is the length of a side. These formulas are the same as the ones used for the volume and surface area of a rectangular prism, but simplified since all three quantities (length, width, and height) are the same.

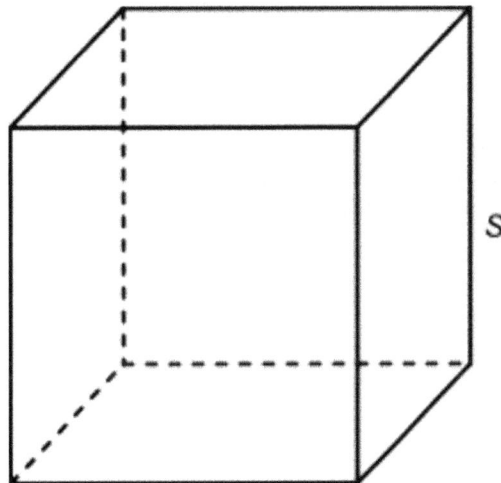

Review Video: <u>Volume and Surface Area of a Cube</u>
Visit mometrix.com/academy and enter code: 664455

The volume of a cylinder can be calculated by the formula $V = \pi r^2 h$, where r is the radius, and h is the height. The surface area of a cylinder can be found by the formula $SA = 2\pi r^2 + 2\pi rh$. The first term is the base area multiplied by two, and the second term is the perimeter of the base multiplied by the height.

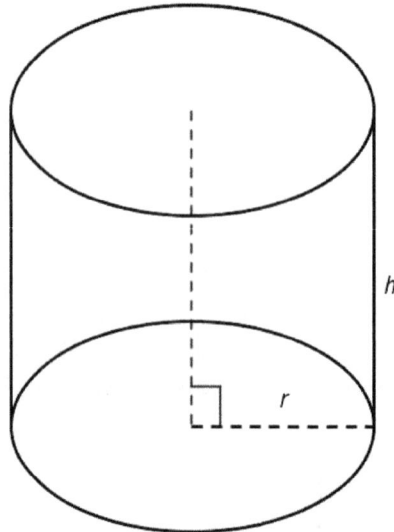

Review Video: <u>Volume and Surface Area of a Right Circular Cylinder</u>
Visit mometrix.com/academy and enter code: 226463

Trigonometry

Defined and Reciprocal Functions

The tangent function is defined as the ratio of the sine to the cosine:

Tangent (tan):

$$\tan x = \frac{\sin x}{\cos x}$$

To take the reciprocal of a number means to place that number as the denominator of a fraction with a numerator of 1. The reciprocal functions are thus defined quite simply.

Cosecant (csc):

$$\csc x = \frac{1}{\sin x}$$

Secant (sec):

$$\sec x = \frac{1}{\cos x}$$

Cotangent (cot):

$$\cot x = \frac{1}{\tan x}$$

It is important to know these reciprocal functions, but they are not as commonly used as the three basic functions.

Inverse Functions

Each of the trigonometric functions accepts an angular measure, either degrees or radians, and gives a numerical value as the output. The inverse functions do the opposite; they accept a numerical value and give an angular measure as the output. The inverse sine, or arcsine, commonly written as either $\sin^{-1} x$ or $\arcsin x$, gives the angle whose sine is x. Similarly:

The inverse of $\cos x$ is written as $\cos^{-1} x$ or $\arccos x$ and means the angle whose cosine is x.

The inverse of $\tan x$ is written as $\tan^{-1} x$ or $\arctan x$ and means the angle whose tangent is x.

The inverse of $\csc x$ is written as $\csc^{-1} x$ or $\operatorname{arccsc} x$ and means the angle whose cosecant is x.

The inverse of $\sec x$ is written as $\sec^{-1} x$ or $\operatorname{arcsec} x$ and means the angle whose secant is x.

The inverse of $\cot x$ is written as $\cot^{-1} x$ or $\operatorname{arccot} x$ and means the angle whose cotangent is x.

Important Note About Solving Trigonometric Equations

When solving for an angle with a known trigonometric value, you must consider the sign and include all angles with that value. Your calculator will probably only give one value as an answer, typically in the following ranges:

For the inverse sine function, $\left[-\frac{\pi}{2}, \frac{\pi}{2}\right]$ or [-90°, 90°]

For the inverse cosine function, [0, π] or [0°, 180°]

For the inverse tangent function, $\left[-\frac{\pi}{2},\frac{\pi}{2}\right]$ or [−90°, 90°]

It is important to determine if there is another angle in a different quadrant that also satisfies the problem. To do this, find the other quadrant(s) with the same sign for that trigonometric function and find the angle that has the same reference angle. Then check whether this angle is also a solution.

In the first quadrant, all six trigonometric functions are positive (sin, cos, tan, csc, sec, cot).

In the second quadrant, sin and csc are positive.

In the third quadrant, tan and cot are positive.

In the fourth quadrant, cos and sec are positive.

If you remember the phrase, "ALL Students Take Classes," you will be able to remember the sign of each trigonometric function in each quadrant. ALL represents all the signs in the first quadrant. The "S" in "Students" represents the sine function and its reciprocal in the second quadrant. The "T" in "Take" represents the tangent function and its reciprocal in the third quadrant. The "C" in "Classes" represents the cosine function and its reciprocal.

TRIGONOMETRIC IDENTITIES
SUM AND DIFFERENCE
To find the sine, cosine, or tangent of the sum or difference of two angles, use one of the following formulas:

$$\sin(\alpha \pm \beta) = \sin\alpha\cos\beta \pm \cos\alpha\sin\beta$$

$$\cos(\alpha \pm \beta) = \cos\alpha\cos\beta \mp \sin\alpha\sin\beta$$

$$\tan(\alpha \pm \beta) = \frac{\tan\alpha \pm \tan\beta}{1 \mp \tan\alpha\tan\beta}$$

where α and β are two angles with known sine, cosine, or tangent values as needed.

HALF ANGLE
To find the sine or cosine of half of a known angle, use the following formulas:

$$\sin\frac{\theta}{2} = \pm\sqrt{\frac{1-\cos\theta}{2}}$$

$$\cos\frac{\theta}{2} = \pm\sqrt{\frac{1+\cos\theta}{2}}$$

where θ is an angle with a known exact cosine value.

To determine the sine of the answer, you must notice the quadrant the given angle is in and apply the correct sign for the trigonometric function you are using. If you need to find the exact sine or cosine of an angle that you do not know, such as sine 22.5°, you can rewrite the given angle as a half angle, such as sine $\frac{45°}{2}$, and use the formula above.

To find the tangent or cotangent of half of a known angle, use the following formulas:

$$\tan\frac{\theta}{2} = \frac{\sin\theta}{1+\cos\theta}$$
$$\cot\frac{\theta}{2} = \frac{\sin\theta}{1-\cos\theta}$$

where θ is an angle with known exact sine and cosine values. These formulas will work for finding the tangent or cotangent of half of any angle unless the cosine of θ happens to make the denominator of the identity equal to 0.

DOUBLE ANGLES

In each case, use one of the Double Angle Formulas.

To find the sine or cosine of twice a known angle, use one of the following formulas:

$$\sin(2\theta) = 2\sin\theta\cos\theta$$
$$\cos(2\theta) = \cos^2\theta - \sin^2\theta \text{ or}$$
$$\cos(2\theta) = 2\cos^2\theta - 1 \text{ or}$$
$$\cos(2\theta) = 1 - 2\sin^2\theta$$

To find the tangent or cotangent of twice a known angle, use the formulas:

$$\tan(2\theta) = \frac{2\tan\theta}{1-\tan^2\theta}$$
$$\cot(2\theta) = \frac{\cot\theta - \tan\theta}{2}$$

In each case, θ is an angle with known exact sine, cosine, tangent, and cotangent values.

PRODUCTS

To find the product of the sines and cosines of two different angles, use one of the following formulas:

$$\sin\alpha\sin\beta = \frac{1}{2}[\cos(\alpha - \beta) - \cos(\alpha + \beta)]$$

$$\cos\alpha\cos\beta = \frac{1}{2}[\cos(\alpha + \beta) + \cos(\alpha - \beta)]$$

$$\sin\alpha\cos\beta = \frac{1}{2}[\sin(\alpha + \beta) + \sin(\alpha - \beta)]$$

$$\cos\alpha\sin\beta - \frac{1}{2}[\sin(\alpha + \beta) - \sin(\alpha - \beta)]$$

where α and β are two unique angles.

COMPLEMENTARY

The trigonometric cofunction identities use the trigonometric relationships of complementary angles (angles whose sum is 90°). These are:

$$\cos x = \sin(90° - x)$$

29

$$\csc x = \sec(90° - x)$$

$$\cot x = \tan(90° - x)$$

PYTHAGOREAN

The Pythagorean Theorem states that $a^2 + b^2 = c^2$ for all right triangles. The trigonometric identity that derives from this principle is stated in this way:

$$\sin^2 \theta + \cos^2 \theta = 1$$

Dividing each term by either $\sin^2 \theta$ or $\cos^2 \theta$ yields two other identities, respectively:

$$1 + \cot^2 \theta = \csc^2 \theta$$

$$\tan^2 \theta + 1 = \sec^2 \theta$$

UNIT CIRCLE

A unit circle is a circle with a radius of 1 that has its center at the origin. The equation of the unit circle is $x^2 + y^2 = 1$. Notice that this is an abbreviated version of the standard equation of a circle. Because the center is the point $(0, 0)$, the values of h and k in the general equation are equal to zero and the equation simplifies to this form.

Standard Position is the position of an angle of measure θ whose vertex is at the origin, the initial side crosses the unit circle at the point $(1, 0)$, and the terminal side crosses the unit circle at some other point (a, b). In the standard position, $\sin \theta = b$, $\cos \theta = a$, and $\tan \theta = \frac{b}{a}$.

Rectangular coordinates are those that lie on the square grids of the Cartesian plane. They should be quite familiar to you. The polar coordinate system is based on a circular graph, rather than the square grid of the Cartesian system. Points in the polar coordinate system are in the format (r, θ), where r is the distance from the origin (think radius of the circle) and θ is the smallest positive angle (moving counterclockwise around the circle) made with the positive horizontal axis.

To convert a point from rectangular (x, y) format to polar (r, θ) format, use the formula (x, y) to $(r, \theta) \Rightarrow r = \sqrt{x^2 + y^2}; \theta = \arctan\frac{y}{x}$ when $x \neq 0$.

If x is positive, use the positive square root value for r. If x is negative, use the negative square root value for r.

If x = 0, use the following rules:

If x = 0 and y = 0, then $\theta = 0$

If x = 0 and y > 0, then $\theta = \frac{\pi}{2}$

If x = 0 and y < 0, then $\theta = \frac{3\pi}{2}$

To convert a point from polar (r, θ) format to rectangular (x, y) format, use the formula (r, θ) to $(x, y) \Rightarrow x = r \cos \theta \; ; y = r \sin \theta$.

> **Review Video: Unit Circle**
> Visit mometrix.com/academy and enter code: 333922

Statistics

MEASURES OF CENTRAL TENDENCY

A **measure of central tendency** is a statistical value that gives a reasonable estimate for the center of a group of data. There are several different ways to measure central tendency. Each one has a unique way it is calculated, and each one gives a slightly different perspective on the data set. Whenever you give a measure of central tendency, always make sure the units are the same. If the data has different units, such as hours, minutes, and seconds, convert all the data to the same unit, and use the same unit in the measure of central tendency. If no units are given in the data, do not give units for the measure of central tendency.

MEAN

The statistical mean of a group of data is the same as the arithmetic average of that group. To find the mean of a set of data, first convert each value to the same units, if necessary. Then find the sum of all the values, and count the total number of data values, making sure you take into consideration each individual value. If a value appears more than once, count it more than once. Divide the sum of the values by the total number of values and apply the units, if any. Note that the mean does not have to be one of the data values in the set, and may not divide evenly.

$$\text{mean} = \frac{\text{sum of the data values}}{\text{quantity of data values}}$$

While the mean is relatively easy to calculate and averages are understood by most people, the mean can be very misleading if it is used as the sole measure of central tendency. If the data set has outliers (data values that are unusually high or unusually low compared to the rest of the data values), the mean can be very distorted, especially if the data set has a small number of values. If unusually high values are countered with unusually low values, the mean is not affected as much. For example, if five of twenty students in a class get a 100 on a test, but the other 15 students have an average of 60 on the same test, the class average would appear as 70. Whenever the mean is skewed by outliers, it is always a good idea to include the median as an alternate measure of central tendency.

MEDIAN

The **statistical median** is the value in the middle of the set of data. To find the median, list all data values in order from smallest to largest or from largest to smallest. Any value that is repeated in the set must be listed the number of times it appears. If there is an odd number of data values, the median is the value in the middle of the list. If there is an even number of data values, the median is the arithmetic mean of the two middle values.

MODE

The **statistical mode** is the data value that occurs the greatest number of times in the data set. It is possible to have exactly one mode, more than one mode, or no mode. To find the mode of a set of data, arrange the data like you do to find the median (all values in order, listing all multiples of data values). Count the number of times each value appears in the data set. If all values appear an equal number of times, there is no mode. If one value appears more than any other value, that value is the mode. If two or more values appear the same number of times, but there are other values that appear fewer times and no values that appear more times, all of those values are the modes.

DISADVANTAGES OF USING MEDIAN OR MODE AS AN ONLY MEASURE OF CENTRAL TENDENCY

The main disadvantage of using the median as a measure of central tendency is that is relies solely on a value's relative size as compared to the other values in the set. When the individual values in a set of data are evenly dispersed, the median can be an accurate tool. However, if there is a group of rather large values or a group of rather small values that are not offset by a different group of values, the information that can be inferred from the median may not be accurate because the distribution of values is skewed. The main disadvantage of the mode is that the values of the other data in the set have no bearing on the mode. The mode may be the largest value, the smallest value, or a value anywhere in between in the set. The mode only tells which value or values, if any, occurred the greatest number of times. It does not give any suggestions about the remaining values in the set.

MEASURES OF DISPERSION

A **measure of dispersion** is a single value that helps to interpret the measure of central tendency by providing more information about how the data values in the set are distributed. The measure of dispersion helps to eliminate or reduce the disadvantages of using the mean, median, or mode as a single measure of central tendency and gives a more accurate picture of the data set as a whole. To have a measure of dispersion, you must know or calculate the range, standard deviation, or variance of the data set.

RANGE

The **range** of a set of data is the difference between the greatest and lowest values of the data in the set. To calculate the range, first make sure the units for all data values are the same, and then identify the highest and lowest values. Write the answer with the same units as the data values that were used to do the calculations.

> **Review Video: Statistical Range**
> Visit mometrix.com/academy and enter code: 778541

STANDARD DEVIATION

Standard deviation is a measure of dispersion that compares all the data values in the set to the mean of the set to give a more accurate picture. To find the standard deviation of a sample, use the following formula:

$$s = \sqrt{\frac{\sum_{i=1}^{n}(x_i - \bar{x})^2}{n-1}}$$

Note that s is the standard deviation of a sample, x_i represents the individual values in the data set, $\bar{x}$ is the mean of the data values in the set, and n is the number of data values in the set. The higher the value of the standard deviation, the greater the variance of the data values from the mean. The units associated with the standard deviation are the same as the units of the data values.

> **Review Video: Standard Deviation**
> Visit mometrix.com/academy and enter code: 419469

Variance

The Variance of a population, or just variance, is the square of the standard deviation of that population. While the mean of a set of data gives the average of the set and gives information about where a specific data value lies in relation to the average, the variance of the population gives information about the degree to which the data values are spread out and tell you how close an individual value is to the average compared to the other values. The units associated with variance are the same as the units of the data values.

Population and Parameter

In statistics, the Population is the entire collection of people, plants, etc., that data can be collected from. For example, a study to determine how well students in the area schools perform on a standardized test would have a population of all the students enrolled in those schools, although a study may include just a small sample of students from each school. A Parameter is a numerical value that gives information about the population, such as the mean, median, mode, or standard deviation. Remember that the symbol for the mean of a population is μ and the symbol for the standard deviation of a population is σ.

Sample and Statistic

A Sample is a portion of the entire population. Whereas a parameter helped describe the population, a Statistic is a numerical value that gives information about the sample, such as mean, median, mode, or standard deviation. Keep in mind that the symbols for mean and standard deviation are different when they are referring to a sample rather than the entire population. For a sample, the symbol for mean is $\bar{x}$ and the symbol for standard deviation is s. The mean and standard deviation of a sample may or may not be identical to that of the entire population due to a sample only being a subset of the population. However, if the sample is random and large enough, statistically significant values can be attained. Samples are generally used when the population is too large to justify including every element or when acquiring data for the entire population is impossible.

Inferential Statistics

There are two types of statistics in common use. Descriptive statistics are those used to describe population data. For example, the mean, the median, and range are all descriptive statistics of a data set. For a given set of data, one can calculate the mean of the sample data, but this does not give any information about whether this mean is what is to be expected or what the data can tell us about the population. Inferential statistics are statistical tools that can be used to infer or draw conclusions about the data set based upon a hypothesis. An example from safety management is to employ a survey of personal protective use among factories owned by the same company in different cities. If there are differences observed in the average percentage of workers in compliance with the policy, is this statistically significant, or just a part of natural variation? We can use inferential statistics to explore whether this is statistically significant. This type of statistics is often seen in political polls, where a sample of the population is questioned about a particular topic or politician to gain an understanding about the attitudes of the entire population of the country. Often, exit polls are conducted on election days using this method. Inferential statistics can have a large margin of error if you do not have a valid sample. Statistical values calculated from various samples of the same size make up the sampling distribution. For example, if several samples of identical size are randomly selected from a large population and then the mean of each sample is calculated, the distribution of values of the means would be a Sampling Distribution.

EVENT

An event, represented by the variable E, is a portion of a sample space. It may be one outcome or a group of outcomes from the same sample space. If an event occurs, then the test or experiment will generate an outcome that satisfies the requirement of that event. For example, given a standard deck of 52 playing cards as the sample space, and defining the event as the collection of face cards, then the event will occur if the card drawn is a J, Q, or K. If any other card is drawn, the event is said to have not occurred.

PROBABILITY

Probability is a branch of statistics that deals with the likelihood of something taking place. One classic example is a coin toss. There are only two possible results: heads or tails. The likelihood, or probability, that the coin will land as heads is 1 out of 2 (1/2, 0.5, 50%). Tails has the same probability. Another common example is a 6-sided die roll. The probability of any given number coming up is 1 out of 6.

PROBABILITY MEASURE

For every sample space, each possible outcome has a specific likelihood, or probability, that it will occur. The probability measure, also called the distribution, is a function that assigns a real number probability, from zero to one, to each outcome. For a probability measure to be accurate, every outcome must have a real number probability measure that is greater than or equal to zero and less than or equal to one. Also, the probability measure of the sample space must equal one, and the probability measure of the union of multiple outcomes must equal the sum of the individual probability measures.

PROBABILITY OF AN EVENT

Probabilities of events are expressed as real numbers from zero to one. They give a numerical value to the chance that a particular event will occur. The probability of an event occurring is the sum of the probabilities of the individual elements of that event. For example, in a standard deck of 52 playing cards as the sample space and the collection of face cards as the event, the probability of drawing a specific face card is $\frac{1}{52} = 0.019$, but the probability of drawing any one of the twelve face cards is $12(0.019) = 0.228$. Note that rounding of numbers can generate different results. If you multiplied 12 by the fraction $\frac{1}{52}$ before converting to a decimal, you would get the answer $\frac{12}{52} = 0.231$.

LIKELIHOOD OF OUTCOMES

The likelihood or probability of an outcome occurring, is given by the formula

$$P(E) = \frac{\text{Number of acceptable outcomes}}{\text{Number of possible outcomes}}$$

where $P(E)$ is the probability of an event E occurring, and each outcome is just as likely to occur as any other outcome. If each outcome has the same probability of occurring as every other possible outcome, the outcomes are said to be equally likely to occur. The total number of possible outcomes in the event must be less than or equal to the total number of possible outcomes in the sample space. If the two are equal, then the event is certain to occur and the probability is 1. If the number of outcomes that satisfy the event is zero, then the event is impossible and the probability is 0.

DETERMINING THE OUTCOME

IN A SIMPLE SAMPLE SPACE

For a simple sample space, possible outcomes may be determined by using a tree diagram or an organized chart. In either case, you can easily draw or list out the possible outcomes. For example, to determine all the possible ways three objects can be ordered, you can draw a tree diagram:

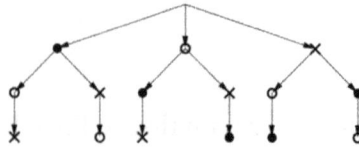

You can also make a chart to list all the possibilities:

First object	Second object	Third object
•	X	O
•	O	X
O	•	X
O	X	•
X	•	O
X	O	•

Either way, you can easily see there are six possible ways the three objects can be ordered.

IN A LESS STRAIGHTFORWARD SAMPLE SPACE

When the test on a given sample space does not lend itself to a tree diagram or organized chart, you can use other methods, such as the multiplication principle, permutations, or combinations, to determine the total number of possible outcomes. Each of these may also be used for simple sample spaces as well, although tree diagrams or charts may be faster in those situations. The multiplication rule states that the probability of two outcomes occurring simultaneously is the product of their individual probabilities. Permutations are outcomes in which each element must occur in a specific order. Combinations are outcomes in which the elements may be arranged in any order.

PERMUTATION AND COMBINATION TO CALCULATE THE NUMBER OF OUTCOMES

When trying to calculate the probability of an event using the $\frac{\text{desired outcomes}}{\text{total outcomes}}$ formula, you may frequently find that there are too many outcomes to individually count them. Permutation and combination formulas offer a shortcut to counting outcomes. A permutation is an arrangement of a specific number of a set of objects in a specific order. The number of permutations of r items given a set of n items can be calculated as $_nP_r = \frac{n!}{(n-r)!}$. Combinations are similar to permutations, except there are no restrictions regarding the order of the elements. While ABC is considered a different permutation than BCA, ABC and BCA are considered the same combination. The number of combinations of r items given a set of n items can be calculated as $_nC_r = \frac{n!}{r!(n-r)!}$ or $_nC_r = \frac{nP_r}{r!}$.

Example: Suppose you want to calculate how many different 5-card hands can be drawn from a deck of 52 cards. This is a combination since the order of the cards in a hand does not matter. There are 52 cards available, and 5 to be selected. Thus, the number of different hands is $_{52}C_5 = \frac{52!}{5! \times 47!} = 2{,}598{,}960$.

ADDITION RULE FOR PROBABILITY

The addition rule for probability is used for finding the probability of a compound event. Use the formula $P(A \text{ or } B) = P(A) + P(B) - P(A \text{ and } B)$, where $P(A \text{ and } B)$ is the probability of both events occurring to find the probability of a compound event. The probability of both events occurring at the same time must be subtracted to eliminate any overlap in the first two probabilities.

MULTIPLICATION RULE FOR PROBABILITY

The multiplication rule can be used to find the probability of two independent events occurring using the formula $P(A \text{ and } B) = P(A) \times P(B)$, where $P(A \text{ and } B)$ is the probability of two independent events occurring, $P(A)$ is the probability of the first event occurring, and $P(B)$ is the probability of the second event occurring. The multiplication rule can also be used to find the probability of two dependent events occurring using the formula $P(A \text{ and } B) = P(A) \times P(B|A)$, where $P(A \text{ and } B)$ is the probability of two dependent events occurring and $P(B|A)$ is the probability of the second event occurring after the first event has already occurred. Before using the multiplication rule, you MUST first determine whether the two events are dependent or independent.

MUTUALLY EXCLUSIVE, INDEPENDENT, AND DEPENDENT

If two events have no outcomes in common, they are said to be mutually exclusive. For example, in a standard deck of 52 playing cards, the event of all card suits is mutually exclusive to the event of all card values. If two events have no bearing on each other so that one event occurring has no influence on the probability of another event occurring, the two events are said to be independent. For example, rolling a standard six-sided die multiple times does not change that probability that a particular number will be rolled from one roll to the next. If the outcome of one event does affect the probability of the second event, the two events are said to be dependent. For example, if cards are drawn from a deck, the probability of drawing an ace after an ace has been drawn is different than the probability of drawing an ace if no ace (or no other card, for that matter) has been drawn.

CONDITIONAL PROBABILITY

Conditional probability is the probability of an event occurring once another event has already occurred. Given event A and dependent event B, the probability of event B occurring when event A has already occurred is represented by the notation $P(A|B)$. To find the probability of event B occurring, take into account the fact that event A has already occurred and adjust the total number of possible outcomes. For example, suppose you have ten balls numbered 1–10 and you want ball number 7 to be pulled in two pulls. On the first pull, the probability of getting the 7 is $\frac{1}{10}$ because there is one ball with a 7 on it and 10 balls to choose from. Assuming the first pull did not yield a 7, the probability of pulling a 7 on the second pull is now $\frac{1}{9}$ because there are only 9 balls remaining for the second pull.

PROBABILITY THAT AT LEAST ONE OF SOMETHING WILL OCCUR

Use a **combination of the multiplication** rule and the rule of complements to find the probability that at least one outcome of the element will occur. This is given by the general formula $P(\text{at least one event occurring}) = 1 - P(\text{no outcomes occurring})$. For example, to find the probability that at least one even number will show when a pair of dice is rolled, find the probability that two odd numbers will be rolled (no even numbers) and subtract from one. You can always use a tree diagram or make a chart to list the possible outcomes when the sample space is small, such as in the dice-rolling example, but in most cases it will be much faster to use the multiplication and complement formulas.

> **Review Video: Multiplication Rule**
> Visit mometrix.com/academy and enter code: 782598

EMPIRICAL PROBABILITY

Empirical probability is based on conducting numerous repeated experiments and observations rather than by applying pre-defined formulas to determine the probability of an event occurring. To find the empirical probability of an event, conduct repeated trials (repetitions of the same experiment) and record your results. The empirical probability of an event occurring is the number of times the event occurred in the experiment divided by the total number of trials you conducted to get the number of events. Notice that the total number of trials is used, not the number of unsuccessful trials. A practical application of empirical probability is the insurance industry. There are no set functions that define life span, health, or safety. Insurance companies look at factors from hundreds of thousands of individuals to find patterns that they then use to set the formulas for insurance premiums.

OBJECTIVE PROBABILITY AND SUBJECTIVE PROBABILITY

Objective probability is based on mathematical formulas and documented evidence. Examples of objective probability include raffles or lottery drawings where there is a pre-determined number of possible outcomes and a predetermined number of outcomes that correspond to an event. Other cases of objective probability include probabilities of rolling dice, flipping coins, or drawing cards. Most gambling is based on objective probability.

Subjective probability is based on personal or professional feelings and judgments. Often, there is a lot of guesswork following extensive research. Areas where subjective probability is applicable include sales trends and business expenses. Attractions set admission prices based on subjective probabilities of attendance based on varying admission rates in an effort to maximize their profit.

CONFIDENCE INTERVAL

A confidence interval consists of three components: a statistic, a margin of error, and a confidence level.

The format is sample statistic $\pm$ margin of error with confidence level of XX%.

The margin of error is the square root of the estimate of the variance, and it is calculated from sample data.

When the distribution of the variable is known, the confidence level may be calculated by the area under the probability distribution function (pdf) and between the upper and lower limits of the confidence interval of the variable. This area is listed in the table for the distribution function, for example the standard normal table.

There is no single way of constructing the confidence interval of an unobservable population parameter, Θ. It depends on the statistical variable whose interval is to be estimated and the distribution of that statistical variable (if any exist). The first rule of constructing an interval is that the upper and lower end-points, U and L, are both functions of the statistical variable X. In other words, the confidence interval will be $(L(X), U(X))$. The probability Pr that the confidence interval

$(L(X), U(X))$ includes the unobservable population parameter θ at the $(1 - \alpha)(100\%)$ confidence level is,

$$Pr\big(L(X) < \theta < U(X)\big) = (1 - \alpha).$$

68-95-99.7 RULE

The *68–95–99.7 Rule* describes how a normal distribution of data should appear when compared to the mean. This is also a description of a normal bell curve. According to this rule, 68 percent of the data values in a normally distributed set should fall within one standard deviation of the mean (34 percent above and 34 percent below the mean), 95 percent of the data values should fall within two standard deviations of the mean (47.5 percent above and 47.5 percent below the mean), and 99.7 percent of the data values should fall within three standard deviations of the mean, again, equally distributed on either side of the mean. This means that only 0.3 percent of all data values should fall more than three standard deviations from the mean. On the graph below, the normal curve is centered on the y-axis. The x-axis labels are how many standard deviations away from the center you are.

Therefore, it is easy to see how the 68-95-99.7 rule can apply.

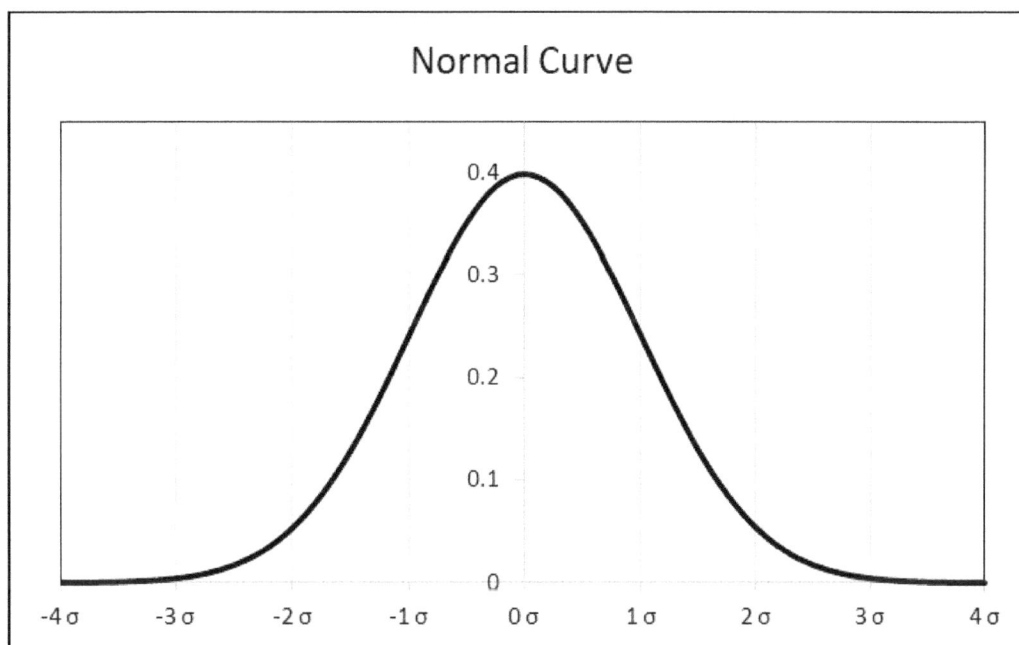

Z-SCORES

A Z-score is an indication of how many standard deviations a given value falls from the mean. To calculate a z-score, use the formula $Z = \frac{x - \mu}{\sigma}$, where x is the data value, μ is the mean of the data set, and σ is the standard deviation of the population. If the z-score is positive, the data value lies above the mean. If the z-score is negative, the data value falls below the mean. These scores are useful in interpreting data such as standardized test scores, where every piece of data in the set has been counted, rather than just a small random sample. In cases where standard deviations are calculated from a random sample of the set, the z-scores will not be as accurate.

Anatomy and Physiology

CELL

The cell is the basic organizational unit of all living things. Each piece within a cell has a function that helps organisms grow and survive. There are many different types of cells, but cells are unique to each type of organism. The one thing that all cells have in common is a membrane, which is comparable to a semi-permeable plastic bag. The membrane is composed of phospholipids. There are also some transport holes, which are proteins that help certain molecules and ions move in and out of the cell. The cell is filled with a fluid called cytoplasm or cytosol.

Within the cell are a variety of organelles, groups of complex molecules that help a cell survive, each with its own unique membrane that has a different chemical makeup from the cell membrane. The larger the cell, the more organelles it will need to live.

CELL STRUCTURAL ORGANIZATION

All organisms, whether plants, animals, fungi, protists, or bacteria, exhibit structural organization on the cellular and organism level. All cells contain **DNA** and **RNA** and can synthesize proteins. All organisms have a highly organized cellular structure. Each cell consists of **nucleic acids**, **cytoplasm**, and a **cell membrane**. Specialized organelles such as **mitochondria** and **chloroplasts** have specific functions within the cell. In single-celled organisms, that single cell contains all of the components necessary for life. In multicellular organisms, cells can become specialized. Different types of cells can have different functions. Life begins as a single cell whether by **asexual** or **sexual reproduction**. Cells are grouped together in **tissues**. Tissues are grouped together in **organs**. Organs are grouped together in **systems**. An **organism** is a complete individual.

NUCLEAR PARTS OF A CELL

- Nucleus (pl. nuclei): This is a small structure that contains the chromosomes and regulates the DNA of a cell. The nucleus is the defining structure of eukaryotic cells, and all eukaryotic cells have a nucleus. The nucleus is responsible for the passing on of genetic traits between generations. The nucleus contains a nuclear envelope, nucleoplasm, a nucleolus, nuclear pores, chromatin, and ribosomes.
- Chromosomes: These are highly condensed, threadlike rods of DNA. Short for deoxyribonucleic acid, DNA is the genetic material that stores information about the plant or animal.
- Chromatin: This consists of the DNA and protein that make up chromosomes.
- Nucleolus: This structure contained within the nucleus consists of protein. It is small, round, does not have a membrane, is involved in protein synthesis, and synthesizes and stores RNA (ribonucleic acid).
- Nuclear envelope: This encloses the structures of the nucleus. It consists of inner and outer membranes made of lipids.
- Nuclear pores: These are involved in the exchange of material between the nucleus and the cytoplasm.
- Nucleoplasm: This is the liquid within the nucleus, and is similar to cytoplasm.

> **Review Video: Chromosomes**
> Visit mometrix.com/academy and enter code: 132083

CELL MEMBRANES

The cell membrane, also referred to as the plasma membrane, is a thin semipermeable membrane of lipids and proteins. The cell membrane isolates the cell from its external environment while still enabling the cell to communicate with that outside environment. It consists of a phospholipid bilayer, or double layer, with the hydrophilic ends of the outer layer facing the external environment, the inner layer facing the inside of the cell, and the hydrophobic ends facing each other. Cholesterol in the cell membrane adds stiffness and flexibility. Glycolipids help the cell to recognize other cells of the organisms. The proteins in the cell membrane help give the cells shape. Special proteins help the cell communicate with its external environment. Other proteins transport molecules across the cell membrane.

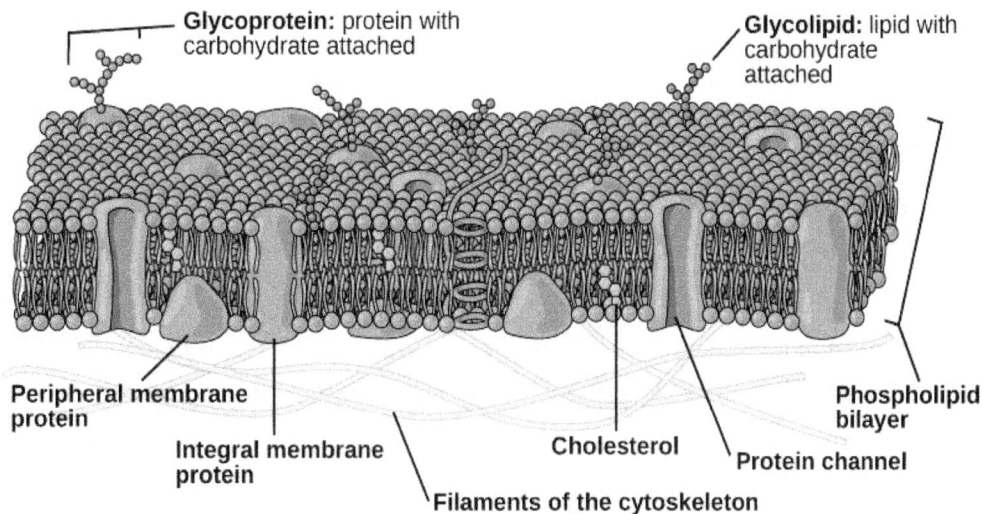

SELECTIVE PERMEABILITY

The cell membrane, or plasma membrane, has selective permeability with regard to size, charge, and solubility. With regard to molecule size, the cell membrane allows only small molecules to diffuse through it. Oxygen and water molecules are small and typically can pass through the cell membrane. The charge of the ions on the cell's surface also either attracts or repels ions. Ions with like charges are repelled, and ions with opposite charges are attracted to the cell's surface. Molecules that are soluble in phospholipids can usually pass through the cell membrane. Many molecules are not able to diffuse the cell membrane, and, if needed, those molecules must be moved through by active transport and vesicles.

ANIMAL TISSUES

Animal tissues may be divided into seven categories:

- Epithelial - Tissue in which cells are joined together tightly. Skin tissue is an example.
- Connective - Connective tissue may be dense, loose or fatty. It protects and binds body parts.
- Cartilage - Cushions and provides structural support for body parts. It has a jelly-like base and is fibrous.
- Blood - Blood transports oxygen to cells and removes wastes. It also carries hormones and defends against disease.
- Bone - Bone is a hard tissue that supports and protects softer tissues and organs. Its marrow produces red blood cells.

- Muscle - Muscle tissue helps support and move the body. The three types of muscle tissue are smooth, cardiac, and skeletal.
- Nervous - Cells called neurons form a network through the body that control responses to changes in the external and internal environment. Some send signals to muscles and glands to trigger responses.

THE THREE PRIMARY BODY PLANES

The **Transverse (or horizontal) plane** divides the patient's body into imaginary upper (superior) and lower (inferior or caudal) halves.

The **Sagittal plane** divides the body, or any body part, vertically into right and left sections. The sagittal plane runs parallel to the midline of the body.

The **Coronal (or frontal) plane** divides the body, or any body structure, vertically into front and back (anterior and posterior) sections. The coronal plane runs vertically through the body at right angles to the midline.

TERMS OF DIRECTION

Medial means nearer to the midline of the body. In anatomical position, the little finger is medial to the thumb.

Lateral is the opposite of medial. It refers to structures further away from the body's midline, at the sides. In anatomical position, the thumb is lateral to the little finger.

Proximal refers to structures closer to the center of the body. The hip is proximal to the knee.

Distal refers to structures further away from the center of the body. The knee is distal to the hip.

Anterior refers to structures in front.

Posterior refers to structures behind.

Cephalad and cephalic are adverbs meaning towards the head. Cranial is the adjective, meaning of the skull.

Caudad is an adverb meaning towards the tail or posterior. Caudal is the adjective, meaning of the hindquarters.

Superior means above, or closer to the head.

Inferior means below, or closer to the feet.

THE INTEGUMENTARY SYSTEM

The integumentary system, which consists of the skin including the sebaceous glands, sweat glands, hair, and nails, serves a variety of functions associated with protection, secretion, and communication. In the functions associated with protection, the integumentary system protects the body from **pathogens** including bacteria, viruses, and chemicals. In the functions associated with secretion, **sebaceous glands** secrete **sebum** (oil) that waterproofs the skin, and **sweat glands** assist with **thermoregulation**. Sweat glands also serve as excretory organs and help rid the body of metabolic waste. In the functions associated with communication, **sensory receptors** distributed throughout the skin send information to the brain regarding pain, touch, pressure, and temperature. In addition to protection, secretion, and communication, the skin manufactures

42

vitamin D with the help of ultraviolet light and can absorb certain chemicals, such as specific medications.

LAYERS OF THE SKIN

The layers of the skin from the surface of the skin inward are the epidermis and dermis. The subcutaneous layer lying below the dermis is also part of the integumentary system. The epidermis is the most superficial layer of the skin. The epidermis, which consists entirely of epithelial cells, does not contain any blood vessels. The deepest portion of the epidermis is the stratum basale, which is a single layer of cells that continually undergo division. As more and more cells are produced, older cells are pushed toward the surface. Most epidermal cells are keratinized. Keratin is a waxy protein that helps to waterproof the skin. As the cells die, they are sloughed off. The dermis lies directly beneath the epidermis. The dermis consists mostly of connective tissue. The dermis contains blood vessels, sensory receptors, hair follicles, sebaceous glands, and sweat glands. The dermis also contains elastin and collagen fibers. The subcutaneous layer or hypodermis is actually not a layer of the skin. The subcutaneous layer consists of connective tissue, which binds the skin to the underlying muscles. Fat deposits in the subcutaneous layer help to cushion and insulate the body.

SKIN AND THERMOREGULATION

The skin is involved in temperature homeostasis or thermoregulation through the activation of the sweat glands. By thermoregulation, the body maintains a stable body temperature as one component of a stable internal environment. The temperature of the body is controlled by a negative feedback system consisting of a receptor, control center, and effector. The receptors are sensory cells located in the dermis of the skin. The control center is the hypothalamus, which is located in the brain. The effectors include the sweat glands, blood vessels, and muscles (shivering). The evaporation of sweat across the surface of the skin cools the body to maintain its tolerance range. Vasodilation of the blood vessels near the surface of the skin also releases heat into the environment to lower body temperature. Shivering is associated with the muscular system.

SEBACEOUS GLANDS AND SWEAT GLANDS

Sebaceous glands and sweat glands are exocrine glands found in the skin. Exocrine glands secrete substances into ducts. In this case, the secretions are through the ducts to the surface of the skin. Sebaceous glands are holocrine glands, which secrete sebum. Sebum is an oily mixture of lipids and proteins. Sebaceous glands are connected to hair follicles and secrete sebum through the hair pore. Sebum inhibits water loss from the skin and protects against bacterial and fungal infections. Sweat glands are either eccrine glands or apocrine glands. Eccrine glands are not connected to hair follicles. They are activated by elevated body temperature. Eccrine glands are located throughout the body and can be found on the forehead, neck, and back. Eccrine glands secrete a salty solution of electrolytes and water containing sodium chloride, potassium, bicarbonate, glucose, and antimicrobial peptides. Eccrine glands are activated as part of the body's thermoregulation. Apocrine glands secrete an oily solution containing fatty acids, triglycerides, and proteins. Apocrine glands are located in the armpits, groin, palms, and soles of the feet. Apocrine glands secrete this oily sweat when a person experiences stress or anxiety. Bacteria feed on apocrine sweat and expel aromatic fatty acids, producing body odor.

THE SKELETAL SYSTEM

The human skeletal system, which consists of 206 bones along with numerous tendons, ligaments, and cartilage, is divided into the axial skeleton and the appendicular skeleton.

The **axial skeleton** consists of 80 bones and includes the vertebral column, rib cage, sternum, skull, and hyoid bone. The **vertebral column** consists of 33 vertebrae classified as cervical vertebrae, thoracic vertebrae, lumbar vertebrae, and sacral vertebrae. The **rib cage** includes 12 paired ribs, 10 pairs of true ribs and two pairs of floating ribs, and the **sternum**, which consists of the manubrium, corpus sterni, and xiphoid process. The **skull** includes the cranium and facial bones. The **ossicles** are bones in the middle ear. The **hyoid bone** provides an attachment point for the tongue muscles. The axial skeleton protects vital organs including the brain, heart, and lungs.

The **appendicular skeleton** consists of 126 bones including the pectoral girdle, pelvic girdle, and appendages. The **pectoral girdle** consists of the scapulae (shoulder blades) and clavicles (collarbones). The **pelvic girdle** attaches to the sacrum at the sacroiliac joint. The upper appendages (arms) include the humerus, radius, ulna, carpals, metacarpals, and phalanges. The lower appendages (legs) include the femur, patella, fibula, tibia, tarsals, metatarsals, and phalanges.

> **Review Video: Skeletal System**
> Visit mometrix.com/academy and enter code: 256447

COMPACT AND SPONGY BONE

Two types of connective bone tissue include compact bone and spongy bone. Compact, or cortical, bone, which consists of tightly packed cells, is strong, dense, and rigid. Running vertically throughout compact bone are the Haversian canals, which are surrounded by concentric circles of bone tissue called lamellae. The spaces between the lamellae are called the lacunae. These lamellae and canals along with their associated arteries, veins, lymph vessels, and nerve endings are referred to collectively as the Haversian system. The Haversian system provides a reservoir for calcium and phosphorus for the blood. Also, bones have a thin outside layer of compact bone, which gives them their characteristic smooth, white appearance. Spongy, or cancellous, bone consists of trabeculae, which are a network of girders with open spaces filled with red bone marrow. Compared to compact bone, spongy bone is lightweight and porous, which helps reduce the bone's overall weight. The red marrow manufactures red and white blood cells. In long bones, the diaphysis consists of compact bone surrounding the marrow cavity and spongy bone containing red marrow in the epiphyses. Bones have varying amounts of compact bone and spongy bone depending on their classification.

FUNCTIONS OF THE SKELETAL SYSTEM

The skeletal system serves many functions including providing structural support, providing movement, providing protection, producing blood cells, and storing substances such as fat and minerals. The skeletal system provides the body with structure and support for the muscles and organs. The axial skeleton transfers the weight from the upper body to the lower appendages. The skeletal system provides movement with joints and the muscular system. Bones provide attachment points for muscles. Joints including hinge joints, ball-and-socket joints, pivot joints, ellipsoid joints, gliding joints, and saddle joints. Each muscle is attached to two bones: the origin and the insertion. The origin remains immobile, and the insertion is the bone that moves as the muscle contracts and relaxes. The skeletal system serves to protect the body. The cranium protects the brain. The vertebrae protect the spinal cord. The rib cage protects the heart and lungs. The pelvis protects the reproductive organs. The red marrow manufactures red and white blood cells. All bone marrow is red at birth, but adults have approximately one-half red bone marrow and one-half yellow bone marrow. Yellow bone marrow stores fat. Also, the skeletal system provides a reservoir to store the minerals calcium and phosphorus.

THE MUSCULAR SYSTEM

The human body has more than 650 skeletal muscles than account for approximately half of a person's weight. Starting with the head and face, the temporalis and masseter move the mandible. The orbicularis oculi closes the eye. The orbicularis oris draws the lips together. The sternocleidomastoids move the head. The trapezius moves the shoulder, and the pectoralis major, deltoid, and latissimus dorsi move the upper arm. The biceps brachii and the triceps brachii move the lower arm. The rectus abdominis, external oblique, and erector spine move the trunk. The external and internal obliques elevate and depress the ribs. The gluteus maximus moves the upper leg. The quadriceps femoris, hamstrings, and sartorius move the lower leg. The gastrocnemius and the soleus extend the foot.

> **Review Video: Muscular System**
> Visit mometrix.com/academy and enter code: 967216

TYPES OF MUSCULAR TISSUE

Smooth muscle tissues are involuntary muscles that are found in the walls of internal organs such as the stomach, intestines, and blood vessels. Smooth muscle tissues, or **visceral tissue,** is nonstriated. Smooth muscle cells are shorter and wider than skeletal muscle fibers. Smooth muscle tissue is also found in sphincters or valves that control the movement of material through openings throughout the body.

Cardiac muscle tissue is involuntary muscle that is found only in the heart. Like skeletal muscle cells, cardiac muscle cells are also striated.

Skeletal muscles are voluntary muscles that work in pairs to move parts of the skeleton. Skeletal muscles are composed of **muscle fibers** (cells) that are bound together in parallel **bundles**. Skeletal muscles are also known as **striated muscle** due to their striped histological appearance under a microscope.

Only skeletal muscle interacts with the skeleton to move the body. When they contract, the muscles transmit **force** to the attached bones. Working together, the muscles and bones act as a system of levers that move around the joints.

SKELETAL MUSCLE CONTRACTION

Skeletal muscles consist of numerous muscle fibers. Each muscle fiber contains a bundle of myofibrils, which are composed of multiple repeating contractile units called sarcomeres. Myofibrils contain two protein microfilaments: a thick filament and a thin filament. The thick filament is composed of the protein myosin. The thin filament is composed of the protein actin. The dark bands (striations) in skeletal muscles are formed when thick and thin filaments overlap. Light bands occur where the thin filament is overlapped. Skeletal muscle attraction occurs when the thin filaments slide over the thick filaments shortening the sarcomere. When an action potential (electrical signal) reaches a muscle fiber, calcium ions are released. According to the sliding filament model of muscle contraction, these calcium ions bind to the myosin and actin, which assists in the binding of the myosin heads of the thick filaments to the actin molecules of the thin filaments. Adenosine triphosphate released from glucose provides the energy necessary for the contraction.

MUSCULAR SYSTEM AND THERMOREGULATION

Thermoregulation or temperature regulation is a homeostatic relationship involving the muscular system. Skeletal muscles and smooth muscles are involved in thermoregulation. If the body temperature drops below acceptable levels, the hypothalamus signals the body's warming mechanisms to initiate. Smooth muscles in the walls of blood vessels in the skin cause the blood vessels to constrict and divert blood into deeper tissues. Skeletal muscles are triggered, and shivering generates heat. When the body temperature rises back to acceptable levels, the hypothalamus signals the body's warming mechanisms to stop. Similarly, if the body temperature rises above acceptable levels, the blood vessels in the skin dilate by means of their smooth muscle tissue. As blood fills the skin's capillaries, heat is radiated away from the body.

THE NERVOUS SYSTEM

The nervous system consists of two major divisions: the central nervous system (CNS) and the peripheral nervous system (PNS). The CNS includes the brain and spinal cord. The brain is the major organ of the nervous system. The brain, which is divided into the cerebrum, cerebellum, and brain stem, controls the entire body including thinking, coordination of skeletal muscle movement, and involuntary actions such as breathing and heart rate. The brain communicates with the rest of the body via the spinal cord. The PNS includes the nerves that branch from the brain and spinal cord. As part of the PNS, 12 pairs of cranial nerves branch off the brain stem. Also extending from the spinal cord are 31 pairs of branching spinal nerves. The PNS includes the somatic nervous system and the autonomic nervous system. The somatic nervous system controls the five senses and the movement of skeletal muscles. The autonomic nervous system includes the sympathetic and parasympathetic nervous system. The sympathetic nervous system deals with stressful or emergency situations, and the parasympathetic nervous system returns the body to normal after stressful or emergency situations and maintains normal functioning.

REFLEX ARC AND STIMULUS

A reflex, the simplest act of the nervous system, is an automatic response without any conscious thought to a stimulus via the reflex arc. The reflex arc is the simplest nerve pathway, which bypasses the brain and is controlled by the spinal cord. For example, in the classic knee-jerk response (patellar tendon reflex), the stimulus is the reflex hammer hitting the tendon, and the response is the muscle contracting, which jerks the foot upward. The stimulus is detected by sensory receptors, and a message is sent along a sensory (afferent) neuron to one or more interneurons in the spinal cord. The interneuron(s) transmit this message to a motor (efferent) neuron, which carries the message to the correct effector (muscle).

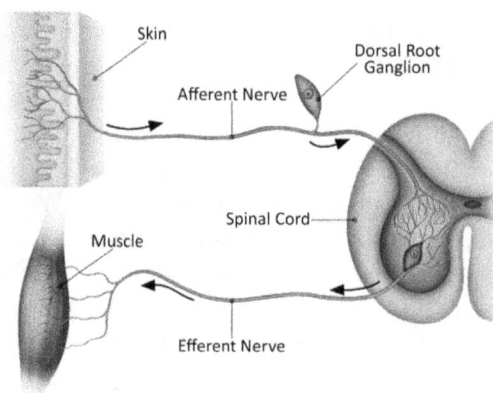

Autonomic Nervous System and Homeostasis

The autonomic nervous system (ANS) maintains homeostasis within the body. In general, the ANS controls the functions of the internal organs, blood vessels, smooth muscle tissues, and glands. This is accomplished through the direction of the hypothalamus, which is located above the midbrain. The hypothalamus controls the ANS through the brain stem. With this direction from the hypothalamus, the ANS helps maintain a stable body environment (homeostasis) by regulating numerous factors including heart rate, breathing rate, body temperature, and blood pH. The ANS consists of two divisions: the sympathetic nervous system and the parasympathetic nervous system. The sympathetic nervous system controls the body's reaction to extreme, stressful, and emergency situations. For example, the sympathetic nervous system increases the heart rate, signals the adrenal glands to secrete adrenaline, triggers the dilation of the pupils, and slows digestion. The parasympathetic nervous system counteracts the effects of the sympathetic nervous system. For example, the parasympathetic nervous system decreases heart rate, signals the adrenal glands to stop secreting adrenaline, constricts the pupils, and returns the digestion process to normal.

Neurons

The three general functional types of neurons are the sensory neurons, motor neurons, and interneurons. Sensory neurons transmit signals to the central nervous system (CNS) from the sensory receptors associated with touch, pain, temperature, hearing, sight, smell, and taste. Motor neurons transmit signals from the CNS to the rest of the body such as by signaling muscles or glands to respond. Interneurons transmit signals between neurons; for example, interneurons receive transmitted signals between sensory neurons and motor neurons. In general, a neuron consists of three basic parts: the cell body, the axon, and many dendrites. The dendrites receive impulses from sensory receptors or interneurons and transmit them toward the cell body. The cell body (soma) contains the nucleus of the neuron. The axon transmits the impulses away from the cell body. The axon is insulated by oligodendrocytes and the myelin sheath with gaps known as the nodes of Ranvier. The axon terminates at the synapse.

The Endocrine System

The endocrine system is responsible for secreting **hormones** and other molecules that help regulate the entire body in both the short and long term. There is a close working relationship between the endocrine and nervous systems. The **hypothalamus** and the **pituitary gland** coordinate to serve as a **neuroendocrine control center**.

Hormone secretion is triggered by a variety of signals, including hormonal signs, chemical reactions, and environmental cues. Only cells with particular **receptors** can benefit from hormonal influence. This is the "key in the lock" model for hormonal action. **Steroid hormones** trigger gene activation and protein synthesis in some target cells. **Protein hormones** change the activity of existing enzymes in target cells. Hormones such as **insulin** work quickly when the body signals an urgent need. Slower-acting hormones afford longer, gradual, and sometimes permanent changes in the body.

> **Review Video: Endocrine System**
> Visit mometrix.com/academy and enter code: 678939

Major Endocrine Glands

1. **Adrenal cortex** - Monitors blood sugar level; helps in lipid and protein metabolism.
2. **Adrenal medulla** - Controls cardiac function; raises blood sugar and controls the size of blood vessels.

3. **Thyroid gland** - Helps regulate metabolism and functions in growth and development.
4. **Parathyroid** - Regulates calcium levels in the blood.
5. **Pancreas islets** - Raises and lowers blood sugar; active in carbohydrate metabolism.
6. **Thymus gland** - Plays a role in immune responses.
7. **Pineal gland** - Has an influence on daily biorhythms and sexual activity.
8. **Pituitary gland** - Plays an important role in growth and development.

Endocrine glands are intimately involved in a myriad of reactions, functions, and secretions that are crucial to the well-being of the body.

THE CIRCULATORY SYSTEM

The **circulatory system** is responsible for the internal transport of substances to and from the cells. The circulatory system consists of the following parts:

- **Blood**: Blood is composed of water, solutes, and other elements in a fluid connective tissue.
- **Blood vessels**: Vessels are tubules of different sizes that transport blood in a closed system to tissues throughout the body.
- **Heart**: The heart is a muscular pump providing the pressure necessary to keep blood flowing throughout the circulatory system.

As the blood moves through the system from larger tubules through smaller ones, the rate slows. The flow of blood in the **capillary beds**, the smallest tubules, is quite slow.

A supplementary system, the **lymph vascular system**, cleans excess fluids and proteins and returns them to the circulatory system.

BLOOD

Blood helps maintain a healthy internal environment in animals by carrying raw materials to cells and removing waste products. It helps stabilize internal pH and hosts cells of the immune system.

An adult human has about five quarts of blood. Blood is composed of **red blood cells, white blood cells**, **platelets**, and **plasma**. Plasma constitutes more than half of the blood volume. It is mostly water and serves as a solvent. Plasma contains plasma proteins, ions, glucose, amino acids, hormones, and dissolved gases. **Platelets** are fragments of stem cells and serve an important function in blood clotting.

Red blood cells transport **oxygen** to cells. Red blood cells form in the bone marrow and can live for about four months. These cells are constantly being replaced by fresh ones, keeping the total number relatively stable. They lack a nucleus.

Part of the immune system, white blood cells defend the body against **infection** and remove wastes. The types of white blood cells include lymphocytes, neutrophils, monocytes, eosinophils, and basophils.

THE HEART

The **heart** is a muscular pump made of cardiac muscle tissue. Heart chamber contraction and relaxation is coordinated by electrical signals from the self-exciting **sinoatrial node** and the **atrioventricular node**. **Atrial contraction** fills the ventricles and **ventricular contraction** forces blood into arteries leaving the heart. This sequence is called the **cardiac cycle**. Valves keep blood moving through the heart in a single direction and prevent any backwash as it flows through its four chambers.

Deoxygenated blood from the body flows through the heart in this order:

9. The **superior vena cava** brings blood from the upper body; the **inferior vena cava** brings blood from the lower body.
10. Right atrium
11. Tricuspid valve (right atrioventricular [AV] valve)
12. Right ventricle
13. Pulmonary valve
14. Left and right pulmonary artery (note: these arteries carry deoxygenated blood)
15. Lungs (where gas exchange occurs)

Oxygenated blood returns to the body through:

16. Left and right pulmonary veins (note: these veins carry oxygenated blood)
17. Left atrium
18. Mitral valve (left atrioventricular [AV] valve)
19. Left ventricle
20. Aortic valve
21. Aortic arch
22. Aorta

The left and right sides of the heart are separated by the septum. The heart has its own circulatory system with its own **coronary arteries**.

BLOOD PRESSURE

Blood pressure is the fluid pressure generated by the cardiac cycle.

Arterial blood pressure functions by transporting oxygen-poor blood into the lungs and oxygen-rich blood to the body tissues. Arteries branch into smaller arterioles which contract and expand based on signals from the body. Arterioles are where adjustments are made in blood delivery to specific areas based on complex communication from body systems.

Capillary beds are diffusion sites for exchanges between blood and interstitial fluid. A capillary has the thinnest wall of any blood vessel, consisting of a single layer of endothelial cells.

Capillaries merge into venules which in turn merge with larger diameter tubules called veins. Veins transport blood from body tissues back to the heart. Valves inside the veins facilitate this transport. The walls of veins are thin and contain smooth muscle and also function as blood volume reserves.

THE RESPIRATORY SYSTEM

The respiratory system can be divided into the upper and lower respiratory system. The **upper respiratory system** includes the nose, nasal cavity, mouth, pharynx, and larynx. The **lower respiratory system** includes the trachea, lungs, and bronchial tree. Alternatively, the components of the respiratory system can be categorized as part of the airway, the lungs, or the respiratory muscles. The **airway** includes the nose, nasal cavity, mouth, pharynx (throat), larynx (voice box), trachea (windpipe), bronchi, and bronchial network. The airway is lined with **cilia** that trap microbes and debris and sweep them back toward the mouth. The **lungs** are structures that house the **bronchi** and bronchial network, which extend into the lungs and terminate in millions of **alveoli** (air sacs). The walls of the alveoli are only one cell thick, allowing for the exchange of gases with the blood capillaries that surround them. The right lung has three lobes. The left lung has only two lobes, leaving room for the heart on the left side of the body. The lungs are surrounded by a **pleural membrane**, which reduces friction between the lungs and walls of the thoracic cavity

49

when breathing. The respiratory muscles include the **diaphragm** and the **intercostal muscles**. The diaphragm is a dome-shaped muscle that separates the thoracic and abdominal cavities; as it contracts, it expands the thoracic cavity which draws air into the lungs. The intercostal muscles are located between the ribs.

> **Review Video: Respiratory System**
> Visit mometrix.com/academy and enter code: 783075

FUNCTIONS OF THE RESPIRATORY SYSTEM

The main function of the respiratory system is to supply the body with **oxygen** and rid the body of **carbon dioxide**. This exchange of gases occurs in millions of tiny **alveoli**, which are surrounded by blood capillaries. The respiratory system also filters air. Air is warmed, moistened, and filtered as it passes through the nasal passages before it reaches the lungs. The respiratory system also allows for speech. As air passes through the throat, it moves through the **larynx** (voice box), which vibrates and produces sound, before it enters the **trachea** (windpipe). Cough production allows foreign particles which have entered the nasal passages or airways to be expelled from the respiratory system. The respiratory system functions in the sense of smell using **chemoreceptors** that are located in the nasal cavity and respond to airborne chemicals. The respiratory system also helps the body maintain acid-base **homeostasis**. Hyperventilation can increase blood pH during **acidosis** (low pH). Slowing breathing during **alkalosis** (high pH) helps lower blood pH.

BREATHING PROCESS

During the breathing process, the diaphragm and the intercostal muscles contract to expand the lungs. During inspiration or inhalation, the diaphragm contracts and moves down, increasing the size of the chest cavity. During expiration or exhalation, the intercostal muscles contract and the ribs expand, increasing the size of the chest cavity. As the volume of the chest cavity increases, the pressure inside the chest cavity decreases (Boyle's law). Because the outside air is under a greater amount of pressure than the air inside the lungs, air rushes into the lungs. When the diaphragm and intercostal muscles relax, the size of the chest cavity decreases, forcing air out of the lungs. The breathing process is controlled by the portion of the brain stem called the medulla oblongata. The medulla oblongata monitors the level of carbon dioxide in the blood and signals the breathing rate to increase when these levels are too high.

THE DIGESTIVE SYSTEM

The digestive system uses the following processes to convert protein, fats, and carbohydrates into usable energy for the body:

- **Movement**: Movement mixes and passes nutrients through the system and eliminates waste.
- **Secretion**: Enzymes, hormones, and other substances necessary for digestion are secreted into the digestive tract.
- **Digestion**: Digestion includes the chemical breakdown of nutrients into smaller units that enter the internal environment.
- **Absorption**: Nutrients pass through plasma membranes into the blood or lymph and then to the body.

The human digestive system consists of the mouth, pharynx, esophagus, stomach, small and large intestine, rectum, and anus. Enzymes and other secretions are infused into the digestive system to assist the absorption and processing of nutrients. The nervous and endocrine systems control the digestive system. Smooth muscle moves the food by peristalsis, contracting and relaxing to move nutrients along.

ROLE OF MOUTH AND STOMACH IN DIGESTION

Digestion begins in the mouth with the chewing and mixing of nutrients with saliva. Only humans and other mammals actually chew their food. Salivary glands are stimulated and secrete saliva. Saliva contains enzymes that initiate the breakdown of starch in digestion. Once swallowed, the food moves down the pharynx into the esophagus en route to the stomach.

The stomach is a flexible, muscular sac. It has three main functions:

1. Mixing and storing food
2. Dissolving and degrading food via secretions
3. Controlling passage of food into the small intestine

Protein digestion begins in the stomach. Stomach acidity helps break down the food and make nutrients available for absorption. Smooth muscle contractions move nutrients into the small intestine where the absorption process begins.

DIGESTION AND THE SMALL INTESTINE

In the digestive process, most nutrients are absorbed in the small intestine. Enzymes from the pancreas, liver, and stomach are transported to the small intestine to aid digestion. These enzymes act on fats, carbohydrates, nucleic acids, and proteins. Bile is a secretion of the liver and is particularly useful in breaking down fats. It is stored in the gall bladder between meals.

By the time food reaches the lining of the small intestine, it has been reduced to small molecules. The lining of the small intestine is covered with villi, tiny absorptive structures that greatly increase the surface area for interaction with chyme. Epithelial cells at the surface of the villi, called microvilli, further increase the ability of the small intestine to serve as the main absorption organ of the digestive tract.

DIGESTION AND THE LARGE INTESTINE

Also called the colon, the large intestine concentrates, mixes, and stores waste material. A little over a meter in length, the colon ascends on the right side of the abdominal cavity, cuts across transversely to the left side, then descends and attaches to the rectum, a short tube for waste disposal.

When the rectal wall is distended by waste material, the nervous system triggers an impulse in the body to expel the waste from the rectum. A muscle sphincter at the end of the anus is stimulated to facilitate the expelling of waste matter.

The speed at which waste moves through the colon is influenced by the volume of fiber and other undigested material present. Without adequate bulk in the diet, it takes longer to move waste along, sometimes with negative effects. Lack of bulk in the diet has been linked to a number of disorders.

DIGESTION AND THE ALIMENTARY CANAL

Digestion occurs in the alimentary canal (gastrointestinal tract), which consists of the mouth, throat (pharynx), esophagus, stomach, small intestine, large intestine, rectum, and anus. Digestion begins in the mouth as food is chewed and mixed with saliva containing enzymes for the digestion of carbohydrates (starches). Peristalsis, involuntary muscle contractions, moves the partially digested food down the esophagus and into the stomach through the lower esophageal sphincter. The stomach, which consists of three layers of smooth muscle lined with a mucous membrane, churns the food with hydrochloric acid (HCl).

The stomach stores the chyme and releases it to the small intestine through the pyloric sphincter. The small intestine consists of three sections: the duodenum, jejunum, and ileum. The duodenum continues breaking down the food with help from the liver, gallbladder, and pancreas. The liver manufactures bile, which is stored in the gallbladder and secreted into the small intestine to aid in the digestion of fats. The pancreas secretes pancreatic juices, which aid in the digestion of carbohydrates, fats, and proteins. The pancreas secretes sodium bicarbonate to neutralize the HCl from the stomach. The jejunum and ileum contain numerous villi for absorption. The large intestine, which houses helpful gut flora, consists of three sections called the ascending colon, transverse colon, and descending colon. The primary function of the large intestine is to absorb water. The rectum stores solid wastes (feces) until they exit the body through the anus.

THE RENAL SYSTEM

The renal system produces and eliminates fluid waste from the body, while maintaining the fluid and pH balance needed for the body to function. It consists mainly of the kidneys, ureters, bladder, and urethra. The mammalian kidney is a bean-shaped organ attached to the body near the peritoneum. The kidney helps to eliminate water and waste from the body. Within the kidney, there are various tubes and capillaries. Substances exit the bloodstream if they are not needed, and those that are needed are reabsorbed. The unnecessary substances are filtered out into the tubules that form urine. From theses tubes, urine flows into the bladder and then out of the body through the urethra.

THE REPRODUCTIVE SYSTEM
MALE REPRODUCTIVE SYSTEM

The functions of the male reproductive system are to produce, maintain, and transfer **sperm** and **semen** into the female reproductive tract and to produce and secrete **male hormones**.

The external structure includes the penis, scrotum, and testes. The **penis**, which contains the **urethra**, can fill with blood and become erect, enabling the deposition of semen and sperm into the female reproductive tract during sexual intercourse. The **scrotum** is a sack of skin and smooth muscle that houses the testes and keeps the testes outside the body wall at a cooler, proper temperature for **spermatogenesis**. The **testes**, or testicles, are the male gonads, which produce sperm and testosterone.

The internal structure includes the epididymis, vas deferens, ejaculatory ducts, urethra, seminal vesicles, prostate gland, and bulbourethral glands. The **epididymis** stores the sperm as it matures. Mature sperm moves from the epididymis through the **vas deferens** to the **ejaculatory duct**. The **seminal vesicles** secrete alkaline fluids with proteins and mucus into the ejaculatory duct also. The **prostate gland** secretes a milky white fluid with proteins and enzymes as part of the semen. The **bulbourethral**, or Cowper's, glands secrete a fluid into the urethra to neutralize the acidity in the urethra, which would damage sperm.

Additionally, the hormones associated with the male reproductive system include **follicle-stimulating hormone (FSH)**, which stimulates spermatogenesis; **luteinizing hormone (LH)**, which stimulates testosterone production; and **testosterone**, which is responsible for the male sex characteristics. FSH and LH are gonadotropins, which stimulate the gonads (male testes and female ovaries). FSH and LH are gonadotropins, which stimulate the gonads (male testes and female ovaries).

FEMALE REPRODUCTIVE SYSTEM

The functions of the female reproductive system are to produce **ova** (oocytes or egg cells), transfer the ova to the **fallopian tubes** for fertilization, receive the sperm from the male, and provide a protective, nourishing environment for the developing **embryo**.

The external portion of the female reproductive system includes the labia majora, labia minora, Bartholin's glands, and clitoris. The **labia majora** and the **labia minora** enclose and protect the vagina. The **Bartholin's glands** secrete a lubricating fluid. The **clitoris** contains erectile tissue and nerve endings for sensual pleasure.

The internal portion of the female reproductive system includes the ovaries, fallopian tubes, uterus, and vagina. The **ovaries**, which are the female gonads, produce the ova and secrete **estrogen** and **progesterone**. The **fallopian tubes** carry the mature egg toward the uterus. Fertilization typically occurs in the fallopian tubes. If fertilized, the egg travels to the **uterus**, where it implants in the uterine wall. The uterus protects and nourishes the developing embryo until birth. The **vagina** is a muscular tube that extends from the **cervix** of the uterus to the outside of the body. The vagina receives the semen and sperm during sexual intercourse and provides a birth canal when needed.

> **Review Video: Reproductive Systems**
> Visit mometrix.com/academy and enter code: 505450

MUTATIONS AND MUTAGENS

Mutations are errors in DNA replication. Mutagens are physical and chemical agents that cause these changes or errors in DNA replication. Mutagens are external factors to an organism. The first mutagens discovered were carcinogens or cancer-causing substances. Other mutagens include ionizing radiation such as ultraviolet radiation, x-rays, and gamma radiation. Viruses and microorganisms that integrate into chromosomes and switch genes on or off causing cancer are mutagens. Mutagens include environmental poisons such as asbestos, coal tars, tobacco, and benzene. Alcohol and diets high in fat have been shown to be mutagenic. Not all mutations are caused by mutagens. Spontaneous mutations can occur in DNA due to molecular decay. Spontaneous errors in DNA replication, repair, and recombination can also cause mutations.

Mutations are changes in DNA sequences. Point mutations are changes in a single nucleotide or at one "point" in a DNA sequence. Three types of point mutations include missense, silent, and nonsense. Missense mutations code for the wrong protein. Silent mutations do not change the function of the protein. Nonsense mutations stop protein synthesis early, resulting in no functioning protein. Deletions and insertions remove and add one or more nucleotides to the DNA sequence, which can remove or add amino acids to the protein, changing the function. Deletions and insertions can also cause a frameshift mutation in which the nucleotides are grouped incorrectly in sets of three. Mutations can also occur on the chromosomal level. For example, an inversion is when a piece of the chromosome inverts or flips its orientation.

Mutations can occur in somatic (body) cells and germ cells (egg and sperm) at any time in an organism's life. Somatic mutations develop after conception and occur in an organism's body cells such as bone cells, liver cells, or brain cells. Somatic mutations cannot be passed on from parent to offspring. The mutation is limited to the specific descendent of the cell in which the mutation occurred. The mutation is not in the other body cells unless they are descendants of the originally mutated cell. Somatic mutations may cause cancer or diseases. Some somatic mutations are silent. Germline mutations are present at conception and occur in an organism's germ cells, which are only egg and sperms cells. Germline mutations may be passed on from parent to offspring. Germline mutations will be present in every cell of an offspring that inherits a germline mutation. Germline mutations may cause diseases. Some germline mutations are silent.

DNA AND RNA

DNA and RNA are both nucleic acids composed of nucleotides made up of a sugar, a base, and a phosphate molecule. DNA and RNA have three of their four bases in common: guanine, cytosine, and adenine. DNA contains the base thymine, but RNA replaces thymine with uracil. DNA is deoxyribonucleic acid. RNA is ribonucleic acid. DNA is located in the nucleus and mitochondria. RNA is found in the nucleus, ribosomes, and cytoplasm. DNA contains the sugar deoxyribose, and RNA contains the sugar ribose. DNA is double stranded, but RNA is single stranded. DNA has the shape of a double helix, but RNA is complexly folded. DNA contains the genetic blueprint and instructions for the cell. RNA carries out those instructions with its various forms. Messenger RNA, mRNA, is a working copy of DNA, and transfer RNA, tRNA, collects the needed amino acids for the ribosomes during the assembling of proteins. Ribosomal RNA, rRNA, forms the structure of the ribosomes.

SUGAR-PHOSPHATE BACKBONE

The DNA molecule consists of two strands in the shape of double helix, which resembles a twisted "ladder." The "rungs" of the ladder consist of complementary base pairs of the nucleotides. The "legs" of the ladder consist of chains of nucleotides joined by the bond between the phosphate and sugar molecules. In DNA, the sugar is deoxyribose. The sugars and phosphates are joined together by covalent bonds. The RNA molecule has one strand instead of two. In RNA, the sugar is ribose. The sugars and phosphates of the nucleotides are joined in the same way.

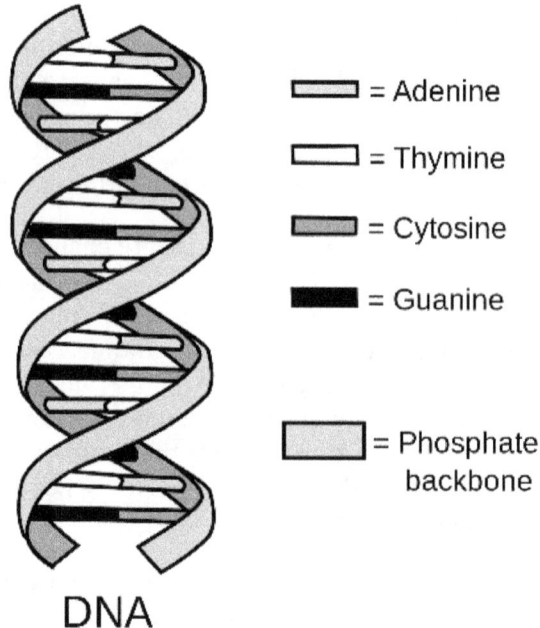

DNA

COMPLEMENTARY BASE PAIRING

According to Chargaff's rule, DNA always has a 1:1 ratio of purine to pyrimidine. The amount of adenine always equals the amount of thymine, and the amount of guanine always equals the amount of cytosine. DNA contains the bases guanine, cytosine, thymine, and adenine. RNA also

54

contains guanine, cytosine, and adenine, but thymine is replaced with uracil. In DNA, adenine always pairs with thymine, and guanine always pairs with cytosine. In RNA, adenine always pairs with uracil, and guanine always pairs with cytosine. The pairs are bonded together with hydrogen bonds.

DNA REPLICATION

DNA replication begins when the double strands of the parent DNA molecule are unwound and unzipped. The enzyme helicase separates the two strands by breaking the hydrogen bonds between the base pairs that make up the rungs of the twisted ladder. These two single strands of DNA are called the replication fork. Each separate DNA strand provides a template for the complementary DNA bases, G with C and A with T. The enzyme DNA polymerase aids in binding the new base pairs together. Short segments of DNA called Okazaki fragments are synthesized with the lagging strand with the aid of RNA primase. At the end of this process, part of the telomere is removed. Then, enzymes check for any errors in the code and make repairs. This results in two daughter DNA molecules each with half of the original DNA molecule that was used as a template.

Physics

EQUILIBRIUM EQUATIONS

If an object is not moving, all the forces on it must be balanced. They are not necessarily equal, but the sum of all the forces acting on the object is zero. This knowledge can be used to calculate missing forces in static situations. For example, if a block rests on the floor without motion, it is at equilibrium. Because the object has some force due to gravity pulling it down, the floor must be

55

opposing the block with an equal, but opposite, force. Two-dimensional force equilibrium says that the sum of all forces in the x- and y-direction is zero, and the sum of all moments is zero:

$$\begin{cases} \sum F_x = 0 \\ \sum F_y = 0 \\ \sum M = 0 \end{cases}$$

CABLES

An ideal cable has no mass, and tension is constant throughout the length. To determine the tension in cables, apply the equilibrium equations. For example, in the diagram below, two cables support a weight of 2000 pounds.

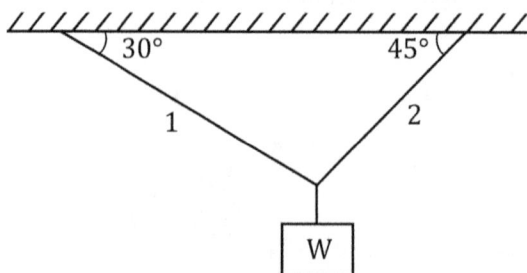

To calculate the tension in each cable, write equilibrium equations for the system. The weight is not accelerating in the x direction, so the sum of the x-components of the cable tensions must be zero.

$$\Sigma F_x = 0 = T_{1_x} + T_{2_x}$$

Once again, there is zero acceleration, so the sum of the weight and the y-components of the cable tensions must be zero.

$$\Sigma F_y = 0 = \text{-2000} + T_{1_y} + T_{2_y}$$

The x- and y-components of the tension in both cables can be solved with trigonometry:

$$T_{1_y} = T_1 \times \sin(30) \quad T_{1_x} = T_1 \times \cos(30)$$

$$T_{2_y} = T_2 \times \sin(45) \quad T_{2_x} = T_2 \times \cos(45)$$

Substituting these equations in for the original equilibrium equations results in:

$$T_1 \cos(30) + T_2 \times \cos(45) = 0$$

$$\text{-2000} + T_1 \times \sin(30) + T_2 \times \sin(45) = 0$$

Now T_1 and T_2 can be calculated by solving for T_1 in the first equation and substituting it in the second equation:

$$T_1 = \frac{T_2 \times \cos(45)}{\cos(30)}$$

$$0 = -2000 + \frac{T_2 \times \cos(45)}{\cos(30)} \times \sin(30) + T_2 \times \sin(45)$$

Therefore, T_2 equals 1793 pounds and T_1 equals 1464 pounds.

PULLEYS

A pulley is a wheel with a grooved rim around which a rope passes. It acts to change the direction of a force applied to the rope, and is chiefly used for lifting heavy weights. An ideal pulley has no mass or friction. In a simple configuration with two equal masses suspended from a single pulley, the force on both rope segments is equal to F, therefore the force on the cable holding the pulley up must be 2×F.

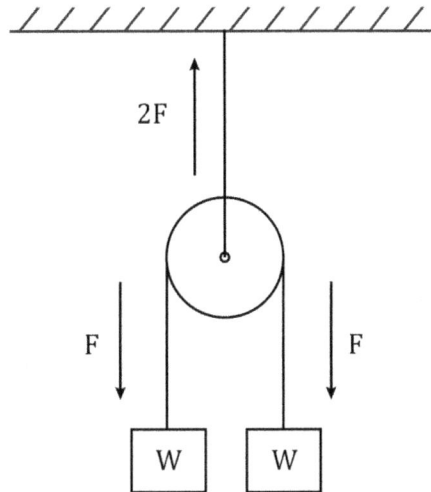

More complex pulley systems can also be analyzed by applying the equations of static equilibrium.

DISTRIBUTED LOADS

Unlike a point load, a distributed load acts upon a length or area of an object. To calculate the effect of a distributed load, it must first be reduced to a resultant load that acts on one point of the length or surface. The magnitude of the resultant force is equal to the area under the curve of the distributed load. The location of the force is at the centroid, or weighted center, of the distributed load.

For example, the beam in the diagram below has a triangle-shaped distributed load on it.

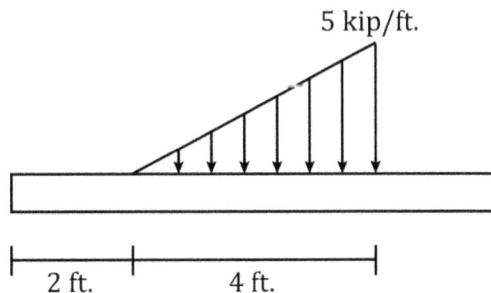

The magnitude of the resultant force can be calculated as such:

$$Area_{triangle} = \frac{1}{2}bh = \frac{1}{2} \times 4 \text{ ft} \times \frac{5 \text{ kips}}{1 \text{ ft}} = 10 \text{ kips}$$

The center of mass of this triangle can be found by plugging the equation of the load into the following equation:

$$\bar{x} = \frac{\int_0^L x \times w(x)\, dx}{\int_0^L w(x)\, dx} = \frac{\int_0^4 x \times \frac{5}{4}x\, dx}{\int_0^4 \frac{5}{4}x\, dx} = 2.66 \text{ ft}$$

Because the load starts two feet down the beam, the actual location of the resultant is at 2+2.66 ft = 4.66 ft.

VELOCITY

There are two types of velocity that are commonly considered in physics: average velocity and instantaneous velocity.

INSTANTANEOUS VELOCITY

In order to obtain the *instantaneous velocity* of an object, we must find its average velocity and then try to decrease Δt as close as possible to zero. As Δt decreases, it approaches what is known as a *limiting value*, bringing the average velocity very close to the instantaneous velocity. Instantaneous velocity is most easily discussed in the context of calculus-based physics.

AVERAGE VELOCITY

f we want to calculate the *average velocity* of an object, we must know two things. First, we must know its displacement, or the distance it has covered. Second, we must know the time it took to cover this distance. Once we have this information, the formula for average velocity is quite simple: $v_{av} = \frac{x_f - x_i}{t_f - t_i}$, where the subscripts i and f denote the initial and final values of the position and time.

In other words, the average velocity is equal to the change in position divided by the change in time. This calculation will indicate the average distance that was covered per unit of time. Average velocity is a vector and will always point in the same direction as the displacement vector (since time is a scalar and always positive).

KINEMATIC EQUATIONS

The phenomenon of constant acceleration allows physicists to construct a number of helpful equations. Perhaps the most fundamental equation of an object's motion is the position equation: $x = \frac{at^2}{2} + v_i t + x_i$. If the object is starting from rest at the origin, this equation reduces to $x = \frac{at^2}{2}$.

The position equation can be rearranged to give the displacement equation: $\Delta x = \frac{at^2}{2} + v_i t$. If the object's acceleration is unknown (but still constant), the position or displacement may be found by the equation $\Delta x = \frac{(v_f + v_i)t}{2}$. If the position of an object is unknown, the velocity may be found by the equation $v = v_i + at$. Similarly, if the time is unknown, the velocity after a given displacement may be found by the equation $v = \sqrt{v_i^2 + 2a\Delta x}$.

ACCELERATION

Acceleration is the change in the velocity of an object. Like velocity, acceleration may be computed as an average or an instantaneous quantity. To calculate average acceleration, we may use this simple equation: $a_{av} = (v_f - V_i)/(t_f - t_i)$, where the subscripts i and f denote the initial and final values of the velocity and time. The so-called instantaneous acceleration of an object can be found by reducing the time component to the limiting value until instantaneous velocity is approached. Acceleration will be expressed in units of distance divided by time squared; for instance, meters per second squared. Like position and velocity, acceleration is a vector quantity and will therefore have both magnitude and direction.

KINETIC ENERGY

The kinetic energy of an object is that quality of its motion that can be related in a qualitative way to the amount of work performed on the object. Kinetic energy can be defined as $KE = \frac{mv^2}{2}$, in which m is the mass of an object and v is the magnitude of its velocity. Kinetic energy cannot be negative, since it depends on the square of velocity. Units for kinetic energy are the same as those for work: joules. Kinetic energy is a scalar quantity.

Changes in kinetic energy occur when a force does work on an object, such that the speed of the object is altered. This change in kinetic energy is equal to the amount of work that is done, and can be expressed as $W = KE_f - KE_i = \Delta KE$. This equation is commonly referred to as the work-kinetic energy theorem. If there are several different forces acting on the object, then W in this equation is simply the total work done by all the forces, or by the net force. This equation can be very helpful in solving some problems that would otherwise rely solely on Newton's laws of motion.

POTENTIAL ENERGY

Potential energy is the amount of energy that can be ascribed to a body or bodies based on configuration. There are a couple of different kinds of potential energy. Gravitational potential energy is the energy associated with the separation of bodies that are attracted to one another gravitationally. Any time you lift an object, you are increasing its gravitational potential energy. Gravitational potential energy can be found by the equation $PE = mgh$, where m is the mass of an object, g is the gravitational acceleration, and h is its height above a reference point, most often the ground.

Another kind of potential energy is elastic potential energy; elastic potential energy is associated with the compression or expansion of an elastic, or spring-like, object. Physicists will often refer to potential energy as being stored within a body, which implies that it could emerge in the future.

> **Review Video: Potential and Kinetic Energy**
> Visit mometrix.com/academy and enter code: 491502

CONVERSION OF ENERGY

There are many different types of energy that exist. These include mechanical, sound, magnetic, electrical, light, heat, and chemical. From the first law of thermodynamics, we know that no energy can be created or destroyed, but it may be converted from one form to another. This does not mean that all forms of energy are useful. Indeed, the second law states that net useful energy decreases in every process that takes place. Most often this occurs when other forms of energy are converted to heat through means such as friction. In these cases, the heat is quickly absorbed into the surroundings and becomes unusable. There are many examples of energy conversion, such as in an automobile. The chemical energy in the gasoline is converted to mechanical energy in the engine.

Subsequently, this mechanical energy is converted to kinetic energy as the car moves. Additionally, the mechanical energy is converted to electrical energy to power the radio, headlights, air conditioner, and other devices. In the radio, electrical energy is converted to sound energy. In the headlights, it is converted to heat and light energy. In the air conditioner, it does work to remove heat energy from the car's interior. It is important to remember that, in all of these processes, a portion of the energy is lost from its intended purpose.

STATIC AND KINETIC FRICTIONAL FORCES

In order to illustrate the concept of friction, let us imagine a book resting on a table. As it sits there, the force of its weight (W) is equal and opposite to the normal force (N). If, however, we were to exert a force (F) on the book, attempting to push it to one side, a frictional force (f) would arise, equal and opposite to our force. This kind of frictional force is known as *static frictional force*. As we increase our force on the book, however, we will eventually cause it to accelerate in the direction of our force. At this point, the frictional force opposing us will be known as *kinetic frictional force*. For the most part, kinetic frictional force is lower than static frictional force, and so the amount of force needed to maintain the movement of the book will be less than that needed to initiate movement. For wheels and spherical objects on a surface, static friction at the point of contact allows them to roll, but there is a frictional force that resists the rolling motion as well, due primarily to deformation effects in the rolling material. This is known as rolling friction, and tends to be much smaller than either static or kinetic friction.

> **Review Video: Friction**
> Visit mometrix.com/academy and enter code: 716782

Chemistry

TEMPERATURE

There are three main scales for measuring temperature. Celsius uses the base reference points of water freezing at 0 degrees and boiling at 100 degrees. Fahrenheit uses the base reference points of water freezing at 32 degrees and boiling at 212 degrees. Celsius and Fahrenheit are both relative temperature scales since they use water as their reference point. The Kelvin temperature scale is an absolute temperature scale. Its zero mark corresponds to absolute zero. Water's freezing and boiling points are 273.15 Kelvin and 373.15 Kelvin, respectively. Where Celsius and Fahrenheit are measured in degrees, Kelvin does not use degree terminology.

- Converting Celsius to Fahrenheit: $°F = \frac{9}{5}°C + 32$
- Converting Fahrenheit to Celsius: $°C = \frac{5}{9}(°F - 32)$
- Converting Celsius to Kelvin: $K = °C + 273.15$
- Converting Kelvin to Celsius: $°C = K - 273.15$

PERIODIC TABLE

The periodic table groups elements with similar chemical properties together. The grouping of elements is based on atomic structure. It shows periodic trends of physical and chemical properties and identifies families of elements with similar properties. It is a common model for organizing and understanding elements. In the periodic table, each element has its own cell that includes varying amounts of information presented in symbol form about the properties of the element. Cells in the table are arranged in rows (periods) and columns (groups or families). At minimum, a cell includes the symbol for the element and its atomic number. The cell for hydrogen, for example, which appears first in the upper left corner, includes an "H" and a "1" above the letter. Elements are ordered by atomic number, left to right, top to bottom.

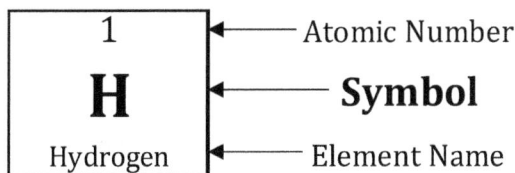

```
┌──────────┐
│    1     │ ◄──── Atomic Number
│          │
│    H     │ ◄──── Symbol
│          │
│ Hydrogen │ ◄──── Element Name
└──────────┘
```

Review Video: The Periodic Table
Visit mometrix.com/academy and enter code: 154828

GROUPS IN THE PERIODIC TABLE

In the periodic table, the groups are the columns numbered 1 through 18 that group elements with similar outer electron shell configurations. Since the configuration of the outer electron shell is one of the primary factors affecting an element's chemical properties, elements within the same group have similar chemical properties. Previous naming conventions for groups have included the use of Roman numerals and upper-case letters. Currently, the periodic table groups are: Group 1, alkali metals; Group 2, alkaline earth metals; Groups 3-12, transition metals; Group 13, boron family; Group 14; carbon family; Group 15, pnictogens; Group 16, chalcogens; Group 17, halogens; Group 18, noble gases.

ADDITIONAL INFORMATION ON THE PERIODIC TABLE

Other information that can be included in each elemental cell includes the atomic weight below the symbol, the element name, colors to organize elements into categories (such as the light pink used for transitional elements and the light blue used for noble gases), colors to indicate the phase of elements (such as red for gas and green for liquid), and line styles around cells to indicate an element's origins (a solid line around the cell indicates a primordial element, a dotted line indicates an element created from decay, and no line indicates that the origins have not yet been discovered). Atomic weight is also known as standard atomic weight or relative atomic mass (not atomic mass), and is defined as the ratio of an average mass of atoms of a specific source of an element to 1/12 of the mass of an atom of carbon-12. Uncertainty may also be included in parenthesis after the atomic weight. Instead of atomic weight, artificial elements may list the most stable isotope in brackets.

PERIODIC TABLE PERIODS AND ELECTRONS

In the periodic table, there are seven periods (rows), and within each period there are blocks that group elements with the same outer electron subshell. The number of electrons in that outer shell determines which group an element belongs to within a given block. Each row's number (1, 2, 3, etc.) corresponds to the highest number electron shell that is in use. For example, row 2 uses only electron shells 1 and 2, while row 7 uses all shells from 1-7.

PERIODIC TABLE AND ATOMIC RADII, IONIC RADII, ELECTRONEGATIVITY

Atomic radii will decrease from left to right across a period (row) on the periodic table. In a group (column), there is an increase in the atomic radii of elements from top to bottom. Ionic radii will be smaller than the atomic radii for metals, but the opposite is true for non-metals. From left to right, electronegativity, or an atom's likeliness of taking another atom's electrons, increases. In a group, electronegativity decreases from top to bottom. Ionization energy or the amount of energy needed to get rid of an atom's outermost electron, increases across a period and decreases down a group. Electron affinity will become more negative across a period but will not change much within a group. The melting point decreases from top to bottom in the metal groups and increases from top to bottom in the non-metal groups.

CHEMICAL EQUATIONS

Chemical equations describe chemical reactions. The reactants are on the left side before the arrow. The products are on the right side after the arrow. The arrow is the mark that points to the reaction or change. The coefficient is the number before the element. This gives the ratio of reactants to products in terms of moles.

The equation for making water from hydrogen and oxygen is $2H_{2(g)} + O_{2(g)} \rightarrow 2H_2O_{(l)}$. The number 2 before hydrogen and water is the coefficient. This means that there are 2 moles of hydrogen and 2 of water. There is 1 mole of oxygen. This does not need to have the number 1 before the symbol for the element. For additional information, the following subscripts are often included to indicate the state of the substance: (g) stands for gas, (l) stands for liquid, (s) stands for solid, and (aq) stands for aqueous. Aqueous means the substance is dissolved in water. Charges are shown by superscript for individual ions, not for ionic compounds. Polyatomic ions are separated by parentheses. This is done so the kind of ion will not be confused with the number of ions.

BALANCING CHEMICAL EQUATIONS

An **unbalanced equation** is one that does not follow the **law of conservation of mass**, which states that matter can only be changed, not created or destroyed. If an equation is unbalanced, the numbers of atoms indicated by the stoichiometric coefficients on each side of the arrow will not be equal. Start by writing the formulas for each species in the reaction. Count the atoms on each side and determine if the number is equal. Coefficients must be whole numbers. Fractional amounts, such as half a molecule, are not possible. Equations can be balanced by adjusting the coefficients of each part of the equation to the smallest possible whole number coefficient. $H_2 + O_2 \rightarrow H_2O$ is an example of an unbalanced equation. The balanced equation is $2H_2 + O_2 \rightarrow 2H_2O$, which indicates that it takes two moles of hydrogen and one of oxygen to produce two moles of water.

SOLUTIONS

A solution is a homogeneous mixture. A mixture is two or more different substances that are mixed together, but not combined chemically. Homogeneous mixtures are those that are uniform in their composition. Solutions consist of a solute (the substance that is dissolved) and a solvent (the substance that does the dissolving). An example is sugar water. The solvent is the water and the solute is the sugar. The intermolecular attraction between the solvent and the solute is called solvation. Hydration refers to solutions in which water is the solvent. Solutions are formed when the forces between the molecules of the solute and the solvent are as strong as the forces holding the solute together. An example is that salt (NaCl) dissolves in water to create a solution. The Na^+ and the Cl^- ions in salt interact with the molecules of water and vice versa to overcome the intramolecular forces of the solute.

PERCENT CONCENTRATIONS

Concentrations can be measured in mole fractions, parts per million or billion, and percent by mass or volume. Percent concentrations can be calculated by mass or by volume by dividing the mass or volume of the solute by the mass or volume of the solution. This quotient is a decimal that can be converted to a percent by multiplying by 100. Many percent concentrations are given as mg/100mL or mg/dL. Other concentrations can be given as mL/mL or mL/dL.

Copyright © Mometrix Media. You have been licensed one copy of this document for personal use only. Any other reproduction or redistribution is strictly prohibited. All rights reserved. This content is provided for test preparation purposes only and does not imply an endorsement by Mometrix of any particular political, scientific, or religious point of view.

MOLARITY

The concentration of a solution is measured in terms of molarity. One molar (M) is equal to a quantity of moles of solute per liter of solution. Adding one mole of a substance to one liter of solution would most likely result in a molarity greater than one. The amount of substance should be measured into a small amount of solution, and then more solution should be added to reach a volume of one liter to ensure accuracy.

THE MOLE AND AVOGADRO'S NUMBER

Atomic mass unit (amu) is the smallest unit of mass, and is equal to 1/12 of the mass of the carbon isotope carbon-12. A mole (mol) is a measurement of molecular weight that is equal to the molecule's amu in grams. For example, carbon has an amu of 12, so a mole of carbon weighs 12 grams. One mole is equal to about 6.0221415×10^{23} elementary entities, which are usually atoms or molecules. This amount is also known as the Avogadro constant or Avogadro's number (NA). Another way to say this is that one mole of a substance is the same as one Avogadro's number of that substance. One mole of chlorine, for example, is 6.0221415×10^{23} chlorine atoms. The charge on one mole of electrons is referred to as a Faraday.

COMMON SOLUTIONS AND DILUTE V. CONCENTRATED SOLUTIONS

A syrup is a solution of water and sugar. A brine is a solution of table salt, or sodium chloride (NaCl), and water. A saline solution is a sterilized concentration of sodium chloride in water. A seltzer is a solution of carbon dioxide in water.

The term dilute is used when there is less solute. Adding more solvent is known as diluting a solution, as is removing a portion of the solute. Concentrated is the term used when there is more solute. Adding more solute makes a solution more concentrated, as does removing a portion of the solvent.

PROPERTIES OF SOLUTIONS

Properties of solutions include: they have a maximum particle size of one nm, they do not separate when allowed to stand or when poured through a fiber filter, they are clear and do not scatter light, and their boiling points increase while their melting points decrease when the amount of solute is increased.

EFFECTS OF TEMPERATURE AND PRESSURE ON SOLUBILITY

Solids tend to dissolve faster when the temperature is increased. Higher temperatures help break bonds through an increase in kinetic energy. Solubility tends to increase for solids being dissolved in water as the temperature approaches 100 °C, but at higher temperatures ionic solutes tend to become less soluble. Gases tend to be less soluble at higher temperatures. When solutions are saturated at high temperatures, the solute will precipitate (return to solid form) and "fall out of the solution" as the solution cools. Melting points can be lowered by using a solvent such as salt on icy roads, which lowers the freezing point of ice. Adding salt to water when making ice cream also lowers the melting point of the water. A solution's melting point is usually lower than the melting point of the solvent alone. Pressure has little effect on the solubility of liquid solutions. In gas solutions, an increase in pressure increases solubility, and vice versa.

POLAR VS. NONPOLAR SOLUTES AND SOLVENTS

For solvation to occur, bonds of similar strength must be broken and formed. Nonpolar substances are usually soluble in nonpolar solvents. Ionic and polar matter is usually soluble in polar solvents. Water is a polar solvent. Oil is nonpolar. Therefore, the saying "oil and water don't mix" is quite true. Heptane (C_7H_{16}) is another nonpolar liquid that is said to be immiscible in water, meaning it can't combine with water. The hydrogen bonds of the water molecules are stronger than the London dispersion forces of the heptane. Polar molecules such as NH_3 (ammonia), SO_2 (sulfur dioxide), and H_2S (hydrogen sulfide) are termed hydrophilic, meaning they readily combine with water. Nonpolar molecules, including the noble gases and other gases such as He (helium), Ne (neon), and CO_2 (carbon dioxide) are termed hydrophobic, meaning they repel or do not readily combine with water. One way to remember this is that "like dissolves like." Polar solvents dissolve polar solutes, while nonpolar solvents dissolve nonpolar solutes.

CHEMICAL REACTIONS

Chemical reactions measured in human time can take place quickly or slowly. They can take a fraction of a second or billions of years. The rates of chemical reactions are determined by how frequently reacting atoms and molecules interact. Rates are also influenced by the temperature and various properties (such as shape) of the reacting materials. Catalysts accelerate chemical reactions, while inhibitors decrease reaction rates. Some types of reactions release energy in the form of heat and light. Some types of reactions involve the transfer of either electrons or hydrogen ions between reacting ions, molecules, or atoms. In other reactions, chemical bonds are broken down by heat or light to form reactive radicals with electrons that will readily form new bonds. Processes such as the formation of ozone and greenhouse gases in the atmosphere and the burning and processing of fossil fuels are controlled by radical reactions.

EFFECT OF TEMPERATURE ON REACTION RATE

The collision theory states that for a chemical reaction to occur, atoms or molecules have to collide with each other with a certain amount of energy. A certain amount of energy is required to breach the activation barrier. Heating a mixture will raise the energy levels of the molecules and the rate of reaction (the time it takes for a reaction to complete). Generally, the rate of reaction is doubled for every 10 degrees Celsius temperature increase. However, the increase needed to double a reaction rate increases as the temperature climbs. This is due to the increase in collision frequency that occurs as the temperature increases. Other factors that can affect the rate of reaction are surface area, concentration, pressure, and the presence of a catalyst.

CATALYSTS

Catalysts, substances that help change the rate of reaction without changing their form, can increase reaction rate by decreasing the number of steps it takes to form products. The mass of the catalyst should be the same at the beginning of the reaction as it is at the end. The activation energy is the minimum amount required to get a reaction started. Activation energy causes particles to collide with sufficient energy to start the reaction. A catalyst enables more particles to react, which lowers the activation energy. Examples of catalysts in reactions are manganese oxide (MnO_2) in the decomposition of hydrogen peroxide, iron in the manufacture of ammonia using the Haber process, and concentrate of sulfuric acid in the nitration of benzene.

COMBINATION AND DECOMPOSITION REACTIONS

Combination, or synthesis, reactions: In a combination reaction, two or more reactants combine to make one product. This can be seen in the equation A + B → AB. These reactions are also known as synthesis or addition reactions. An example is burning hydrogen in air to produce water. The equation is $2H_2$ (g) + O_2 (g) → $2H_2O$ (l). Another example is when water and sulfur trioxide react to form sulfuric acid. The equation is H_2O + SO_3 → H_2SO_4.

Decomposition (or desynthesis, decombination, or deconstruction) **reactions** are chemical reactions whereby a reactant is broken down into two or more products. This can be seen in the equation AB → A + B. These reactions are also called analysis reactions. Decomposition reactions can be viewed as the opposite of combination reactions. Most decomposition reactions are **endothermic,** meaning that heat needs to be added for the chemical reaction to occur. **Thermal decomposition** is caused by heat. **Electrolytic decomposition** is caused by electricity. An example of this type of reaction is the decomposition of water into hydrogen and oxygen gas. The equation is $2H_2O \rightarrow 2H_2 + O_2$.

COMBUSTION

Combustion, or burning, is a sequence of chemical reactions involving fuel and an oxidant that produces heat and sometimes light. There are many types of combustion, such as rapid, slow, complete, turbulent, microgravity, and incomplete. Fuels and oxidants determine the compounds formed by a combustion reaction. For example, when rocket fuel consisting of hydrogen and oxygen combusts, it results in the formation of water vapor. When air and wood burn, resulting compounds include nitrogen, unburned carbon, and carbon compounds. Combustion is an exothermic process, meaning it releases energy. Exothermic energy is commonly released as heat, but can take other forms, such as light, electricity, or sound.

SINGLE AND DOUBLE SUBSTITUTION REACTIONS

Single substitution, displacement, or replacement reactions occur when one reactant is displaced by another to form the final product (A + BC → B + AC). Single substitution reactions can be cationic or anionic. When a piece of copper (Cu) is placed into a solution of silver nitrate ($AgNO_3$), the solution turns blue. The copper appears to be replaced with a silvery-white material. The equation is $2AgNO_3 + Cu \rightarrow Cu(NO_3)_2 + 2Ag$. When this reaction takes place, the copper dissolves and the silver in the silver nitrate solution precipitates (becomes a solid), resulting in copper nitrate and silver. Copper and silver have switched places in the nitrate.

> **Review Video: What is a Single-Replacement Reaction?**
> Visit mometrix.com/academy and enter code: 442975

Double displacement, double replacement, substitution, metathesis, or ion exchange reactions occur when ions or bonds are exchanged by two compounds to form different compounds (AC + BD → AD + BC). An example of this is that silver nitrate and sodium chloride form two different products (silver chloride and sodium nitrate) when they react. The formula for this reaction is $AgNO_3 + NaCl \rightarrow AgCl + NaNO_3$.

COVALENT AND IONIC BONDING

Covalent bonding results from the sharing of electrons between atoms. Atoms seek to fill their valence shell and will share electrons with another atom in order to have a full octet (except hydrogen and helium, which only hold two electrons in their valence shells). Molecular compounds have covalent bonds. Organic compounds such as proteins, carbohydrates, lipids, and nucleic acids are molecular compounds formed by covalent bonds. Methane (CH_4) is a molecular compound in which one carbon atom is covalently bonded to four hydrogen atoms as shown below.

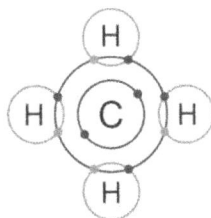

Ionic bonding results from the transfer of electrons between atoms. A cation or positive ion is formed when an atom loses one or more electrons. An anion or negative ion is formed when an atom gains one or more electrons. An ionic bond results from the electrostatic attraction between a cation and an anion. One example of a compound formed by ionic bonds is sodium chloride or NaCl. Sodium (Na) is an alkali metal and tends to form Na+ ions. Chlorine is a halogen and tends to form Cl- ions. The Na+ ion and the Cl- ion are attracted to each other. This electrostatic attraction between these oppositely charged ions is what results in the ionic bond between them.

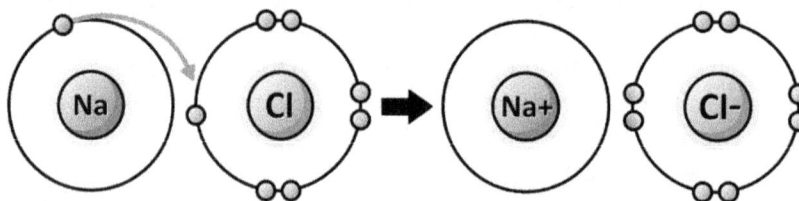

HYDROGEN BONDS

Hydrogen bonds are weaker than covalent and ionic bonds, and refer to the type of attraction in an electronegative atom such as oxygen, fluorine, or nitrogen. Hydrogen bonds can form within a single molecule or between molecules. A water molecule is polar, meaning it is partially positively charged on one end (the hydrogen end) and partially negatively charged on the other (the oxygen end). This is because the hydrogen atoms are arranged around the oxygen atom in a close tetrahedron. Hydrogen is oxidized (its number of electrons is reduced) when it bonds with oxygen to form water. Hydrogen bonds tend not only to be weak but also short-lived. They also tend to be numerous. Hydrogen bonds give water many of its important properties, including its high specific heat and high heat of vaporization, its solvent qualities, its adhesiveness and cohesiveness, its hydrophilic qualities, and its ability to float in its solid form. Hydrogen bonds are also an important component of proteins, nucleic acids, and DNA.

INTERMOLECULAR FORCES

Intermolecular forces are weaker than ionic and covalent bonds. They occur between stable molecules or functional groups of macromolecules. Macromolecules are large molecules that are usually created by polymerization and sometimes distinguished by their lack of covalent bonds. London dispersion force, dipole-dipole interactions, and hydrogen bonding are all examples of intermolecular forces. London dispersion force is also known as instantaneous dipole-induced dipole force because the force is caused by a change in dipole (a separation of the positive and negative charges in an atom). These forces are weak and the attractions are quickly formed and broken. An electron from one atom affects another atom, resulting in a force that dissipates as soon as an electron moves. Dipole-dipole (Keesom) interactions occur within atoms that are already covalently bonded and have permanent dipoles. These atoms have a different amount of electronegativity (attraction of electrons). One atom attracts another, electrostatic forces are generated, and molecules align to increase this attraction.

OXIDATION-REDUCTION REACTIONS

One way to organize chemical reactions is to sort them into two categories: oxidation/reduction reactions (also called redox reactions) and metathesis reactions (which include acid/base reactions). Oxidation/reduction reactions can involve the transfer of one or more electrons, or they can occur as a result of the transfer of oxygen, hydrogen, or halogen atoms. The species that loses electrons is oxidized and is referred to as the reducing agent. The species that gains electrons is reduced and is referred to as the oxidizing agent. The element undergoing oxidation experiences an increase in its oxidation number, while the element undergoing reduction experiences a decrease in its oxidation number. Single replacement reactions are types of oxidation/reduction reactions. In a single replacement reaction, electrons are transferred from one chemical species to another. The transfer of electrons results in changes in the nature and charge of the species.

OXIDATION STATE AND OXIDATION NUMBER

Oxidation state and oxidation number are usually the same number. Even though they have different meanings, they are frequently used interchangeably. Oxidation numbers are Roman numerals in parentheses that are used as part of the naming scheme for inorganic compounds. Oxidation state refers to the hypothetical charge on an atom if all of its bonds are 100 percent ionic. They are integers that can occasionally be fractional numbers. Oxidation state is increased through oxidation (loss of electrons) and decreased through reduction (gain of electrons). The number for an oxidation state refers to a single atom or ion, and is a way to keep track of electrons. When using Lewis diagrams, shared electrons are generally assigned to the more electronegative element. In bonds involving two atoms of the same element, electrons are split between them. Lone pairs of electrons are assigned to the atom they are with.

RULES FOR DETERMINING OXIDATION STATE

Rules for calculating oxidation state include the one that states that the oxidation state is 0 for atoms in elemental form (only one kind of atom is present and its charge is 0). For example, both S_8 and Fe have an oxidation state of 0. For a monatomic ion, the oxidation state is equal to its charge. For example, the oxidation state is -2 for S^{2-} and +3 for Al^{3+}. For all Group 1A (alkali) metals, the oxidation state is +1. It is +2 for all Group 2A (alkaline earth) metals unless they are in elemental form. Hydrogen has an oxidation state of +1 when it is bonded to a nonmetal. It can be -1 when bonded to a metal. Oxygen almost always has an oxidation state of -2, but in peroxides it is -1. There are other exceptions as well. The oxidation state for fluorine is always -1. In a neutral compound, the sum of all atoms or ions must equal zero. In a polyatomic ion, its charge is equal to the sum of all oxidation state numbers.

ACIDS AND BASES
ACIDS

When they are dissolved in aqueous solutions, some properties of acids are that they conduct electricity, change blue litmus paper to red, have a sour taste, react with bases to neutralize them, and react with active metals to free hydrogen. A weak acid is one that does not donate all of its protons or disassociate completely. Strong acids include hydrochloric, hydriodic, hydrobromic, perchloric, nitric, and sulfuric. They ionize completely. Superacids are those that are stronger than 100 percent sulfuric acid. They include fluoroantimonic, magic, and perchloric acids. Acids can be used in pickling, a process used to remove rust and corrosion from metals. They are also used as catalysts in the processing of minerals and the production of salts and fertilizers. Phosphoric acid (H_3PO_4) is added to sodas and other acids are added to foods as preservatives or to add taste.

BASES

When they are dissolved in aqueous solutions, some properties of bases are that they conduct electricity, change red litmus paper to blue, feel slippery, and react with acids to neutralize their properties. A weak base is one that does not completely ionize in an aqueous solution, and usually has a low pH. Strong bases can free protons in very weak acids. Examples of strong bases are hydroxide compounds such as potassium, barium, and lithium hydroxides. Most are in the first and second groups of the periodic table. A superbase is extremely strong compared to sodium hydroxide and cannot be kept in an aqueous solution. Superbases are organized into organic, organometallic, and inorganic classes. Bases are used as insoluble catalysts in heterogeneous reactions and as catalysts in hydrogenation.

Review Video: Properties of Acids and Bases
Visit mometrix.com/academy and enter code: 645283

pH

The **pH**, or potential of hydrogen, is a measurement of the concentration of hydrogen ions in a substance in terms of the number of moles of H^+ per liter of solution. Nearly all substances fall between 0 and 14 on the pH scale. A lower pH indicates a higher H^+ concentration, while a higher pH indicates a lower H^+ concentration.

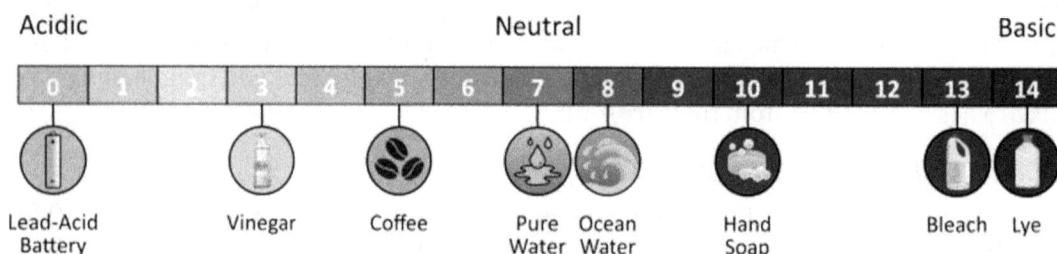

Pure water has a neutral pH, which is 7. Anything with a pH lower than pure water (<7) is considered **acidic**. Anything with a pH higher than pure water (>7) is a **base**. Drain cleaner, soap, baking soda, ammonia, egg whites, and sea water are common bases. Urine, stomach acid, citric acid, vinegar, hydrochloric acid, and battery acid are acids. A **pH indicator** is a substance that acts as a detector of hydrogen or hydronium ions. Such an indicator is **halochromic**, meaning it changes color to indicate that hydrogen or hydronium ions have been detected.

Review Video: Overview of pH Levels
Visit mometrix.com/academy and enter code: 187395

NUCLEAR CHEMISTRY
NUCLEAR REACTIONS

The particles of an atom's nucleus (the protons and neutrons) are bound together by nuclear force, also known as residual strong force. Unlike chemical reactions, which involve electrons, nuclear reactions occur when two nuclei or nuclear particles collide. This results in the release or absorption of energy and products that are different from the initial particles. The energy released in a nuclear reaction can take various forms, including the release of kinetic energy of the product particles and the emission of very high energy photons known as gamma rays. Some energy may also remain in the nucleus. Radioactivity refers to the particles emitted from nuclei as a result of nuclear instability. There are many nuclear isotopes that are unstable and can spontaneously emit some kind of radiation. The most common types of radiation are alpha, beta, and gamma radiation, but there are several other varieties of radioactive decay.

RADIOACTIVE HALF-LIFE AND RADIATION

Radioactive half-life is the time it takes for half of the radioactive nuclei in a sample to undergo radioactive decay. Radioactive decay rates are usually expressed in terms of half-lives. The different types of radioactivity lead to different decay paths, which transmute the nuclei into other chemical elements. Decay products (or daughter nuclides) make radioactive dating possible. Decay chains are a series of decays that result in different products. For example, uranium-238 is often found in granite. Its decay chain includes 14 daughter products. It eventually becomes a stable isotope of lead, which is why lead is often found with deposits of uranium ore. Its first half-life is equivalent to the approximate age of the earth, about 4.5 billion years. One of its products is radon, a radioactive gas. Radiation occurs when energy is emitted by one body and absorbed by another. Nuclear weapons, nuclear reactors, and radioactive substances are all examples of things that involve ionizing radiation. Acoustic and electromagnetic radiation are other types of radiation.

ISOTOPES

The number of protons in an atom determines the element of that atom. For instance, all helium atoms have exactly two protons, and all oxygen atoms have exactly eight protons. If two atoms have the same number of protons, then they are the same element. However, the number of neutrons in two atoms can be different without the atoms being different elements. Isotope is the term used to distinguish between atoms that have the same number of protons but a different number of neutrons. The names of isotopes have the element name with the mass number. Recall that the mass number is the number of protons plus the number of neutrons. For example, carbon-12 refers to an atom that has 6 protons, which makes it carbon, and 6 neutrons. In other words, 6 protons + 6 neutrons = 12. Carbon-13 has six protons and seven neutrons, and carbon-14 has six protons and eight neutrons. Isotopes can also be written with the mass number in superscript before the element symbol. For example, carbon-12 can be written as ^{12}C.

RADIOISOTOPES, RADIOACTIVE DECAY, RADIOACTIVITY

Radioisotopes: Also known as radionuclides or radioactive isotopes, radioisotopes are atoms that have an unstable nucleus. This is a nucleus that has excess energy and the potential to make radiation particles within the nucleus (subatomic particles) or undergo radioactive decay, which can result in the emission of gamma rays. Radionuclides may occur naturally, but can also be artificially produced.

Radioactive decay: This occurs when an unstable atomic nucleus spontaneously loses energy by emitting ionizing particles and radiation. Decay is a form of energy transfer, as energy is lost. It also results in different products. Before decay there is one type of atom, called the parent nuclide. After decay there are one or more different products, called the daughter nuclide(s).

Radioactivity: This refers to particles that are emitted from nuclei as a result of nuclear instability.

STABLE AND RADIOACTIVE ISOTOPES

Stable isotopes: Isotopes that have not been observed to decay are stable, or non-radioactive, isotopes. It is not known whether some stable isotopes may have such long decay times that observing decay is not possible. Currently, 80 elements have one or more stable isotopes. There are 256 known stable isotopes in total. Carbon, for example, has three isotopes. Two (carbon-12 and carbon-13) are stable and one (carbon-14) is radioactive.

Radioactive isotopes: These have unstable nuclei and can undergo spontaneous nuclear reactions, which results in particles or radiation being emitted. It cannot be predicted when a specific nucleus will decay, but large groups of identical nuclei decay at predictable rates. Knowledge about rates of decay can be used to estimate the age of materials that contain radioactive isotopes.

ALPHA, BETA, AND GAMMA RAYS

Ionizing radiation is that which can cause an electron to detach from an atom. It occurs in radioactive reactions and comes in three types: alpha (α), beta (β), and gamma (γ). Alpha rays are positive, beta rays are negative, and gamma rays are neutral. Alpha particles are larger than beta particles and can cause severe damage if ingested. Because of their large mass, however, they can be stopped easily. Even paper can protect against this type of radiation. Beta particles can be beta-minus or beta-plus. Beta-minus particles contain an energetic electron, while beta-plus particles are emitted by positrons and can result in gamma photons. Beta particles can be stopped with thin metal. Gamma rays are a type of high energy electromagnetic radiation consisting of photons. Gamma radiation rids the decaying nucleus of excess energy after it has emitted either alpha or beta radiation. Gamma rays can cause serious damage when absorbed by living tissue, and it takes thick lead to stop them. Alpha, beta, and gamma radiation can also have positive applications.

BIOCHEMISTRY

CARBOHYDRATES

The simple sugars can be grouped into monosaccharides (glucose, fructose, and galactose) and disaccharides. These are both types of carbohydrates. Monosaccharides have one monomer of sugar and disaccharides have two. Monosaccharides (CH_2O) have one carbon for every water molecule. Aldose and ketose are monosaccharides with a carbonyl (=O, double bonded oxygen to carbon) functional group. The difference between aldose and ketose is that the carbonyl group in aldose is connected at an end carbon and the carbonyl group in ketose is connected at a middle carbon. Glucose is a monosaccharide containing six carbons, making it a hexose and an aldose. A disaccharide is formed from two monosaccharides with a glycosidic link. Examples include two glucoses forming a maltose, a glucose and a galactose forming a lactose, and a glucose and a fructose forming a sucrose. A starch is a polysaccharide consisting only of glucose monomers. Examples are amylose, amylopectin, and glycogen.

In glycolysis, glucose is converted into pyruvate and energy stored in ATP bonds is released. Glycolysis can involve various pathways. Various intermediates are produced that are used in other processes, and the pyruvic acid produced by glycolysis can be further used for respiration by the Krebs cycle or in fermentation. Glycolysis occurs in both aerobic and anaerobic organisms. Oxidation of molecules produces reduced coenzymes, such as NADH. The coenzymes relocate hydrogens to the electron transport chain. The proton is transported through the cell membrane and the electron is transported down the chain by proteins. At the end of the chain, water is formed when the final acceptor releases two electrons that combine with oxygen. The protons are pumped back into the cell or organelle by the ATP synthase enzyme, which uses energy produced to add a phosphate to ADP to form ATP. The proton motive force is produced by the protons being moved across the membrane.

Glycolysis can involve different metabolic pathways. The following 10 steps are based on the Embden-Meyerhof pathway, in which glucose is the starting product and pyruvic acid is the final product. Two molecules of ATP and two of NADH are the products of this process. To start, enzymes utilize ATP to form glucose-6-phosphate. The glucose-6 is converted to fructose-6-phosphate. Another ATP molecule and an enzyme are used to convert fructose-6-phosphate to fructose-1,6-disphosphate. Both dihydroxyacetone phosphate (DHAP) and glyceraldehyde-3-phosphate are formed from fructose-1,6-disphosphate. It is during the preceding reactions that energy is conserved or gained. NAD conversions to NADH molecules and phosphate influx result in 1,3-diphosphoglceric acid. Then, two ADP molecules are phosphorylated into ATP molecules, resulting in 3-phosphoglyceric acid, which reforms into 2-phosphoglyceric acid. At this point, water is produced as a product and phosphoenolpyruvic acid is formed. Another set of ADP molecules are phosphorylated into ATP molecules. Pyruvic acid is the end result.

Glycolysis is a general term for the conversion of glucose into pyruvate.

Embden-Meyerhof pathway: This is a type of glycolysis in which one molecule of glucose becomes two ATP and two NADH molecules. Pyruvic acid (two pyruvate molecules) is the end product.

Entner-Doudoroff pathway: This is a type of glycolysis in which one glucose molecule forms into one molecule of ATP and two of NADPH, which are used for other reactions. The end product is two pyruvate molecules.

Pentose Phosphate pathway: Also known as the hexose monophosphate shunt, this is a type of glycolysis in which one glucose molecule produces one ATP and two NADPH molecules. Five carbon sugars are metabolized during this reaction. Glucose is broken down into ribose, ribulose, and xylose, which are used during glycolysis and during the Calvin (or Calvin-Benson) cycle to create nucleotides, nucleic acids, and amino acids.

PROTEINS

Proteins are macromolecules formed from amino acids. They are polypeptides, which consist of many (10 to 100) peptides linked together. The peptide connections are the result of condensation reactions. A condensation reaction results in a loss of water when two molecules are joined together. A hydrolysis reaction is the opposite of a condensation reaction. During hydrolysis, water is added. -H is added to one of the smaller molecules and OH is added to another molecule being formed. A peptide is a compound of two or more amino acids. Amino acids are formed by the partial hydrolysis of protein, which forms an amide bond. This partial hydrolysis involves an amine group and a carboxylic acid. In the carbon chain of amino acids, there is a carboxylic acid group (-COOH), an amine group ($-NH_2$), a central carbon atom between them with an attached hydrogen, and an attached "R" group (side chain), which is different for different amino acids. It is the "R" group that determines the properties of the protein.

Alkyl: This is a nonpolar group that forms hydrophobic amino acids. Amino acids include glycine with a single hydrogen atom R group, alanine with a methyl R group, and valine with an isopropyl R group. Leucine and isoleucine also have alkyl side chains.

Hydroxyl: This is a polar group that forms hydrophilic amino acids such as serine and threonine.

Sulfur: Amino acids in this group include cysteine and methionine.

Carboxylic acid: In this group, a second carboxylic acid group is attached as the R group. This acid group is polar and can be negatively charged when the acidic proton attaches to a water molecule, which leaves a negatively charged carboxylate ion. Amino acids that belong to this group include aspartic acid and glutamic acid.

Amide: The formula for amides is $-CONH_2$. Amino acids belonging to this group include glutamine and asparagine.

Amino: This group includes lysine, arginine, and histidine. The double-bonded nitrogen atom can take a proton to become positively charged.

Aromatic: This group has a ring structure, and includes the amino acids phenylalanine, tyrosine, and tryptophan. Tyrosine is polar, while tryptophan and phenylalanine are nonpolar.

Looped: This group includes proline. Because it is nonpolar, it forms a ring rather than a chain.

LIPIDS

Carbohydrates, proteins, and nucleic acids are groups of macromolecules that are polymers. Lipids are molecules that are soluble in nonpolar solvents, but they are hydrophobic, meaning they do not bond well with water or mix well with water solutions. Lipids have numerous C-H bonds. In this way, they are similar to hydrocarbons (substances consisting only of carbon and hydrogen).The

71

major roles of lipids include energy storage and structural functions. Examples of lipids include fats, phospholipids, steroids, and waxes. Fats are made of long chains of fatty acids (three fatty acids bound to a glycerol). Fatty acids are chains with reduced carbon at one end and a carboxylic acid group at the other. An example is soap, which contains the sodium salts of free fatty acids. Phospholipids are lipids that have a phosphate group rather than a fatty acid. Glycerides are another type of lipid. Examples of glycerides are fat and oil. Glycerides are formed from fatty acids and glycerol (a type of alcohol).

NUCLEIC ACIDS

Nucleic acids are macromolecules that are composed of nucleotides. Hydrolysis is a reaction in which water is broken down into hydrogen cations (H or H^+) and hydroxide anions (OH or OH^-). This is part of the process by which nucleic acids are broken down by enzymes to produce shorter strings of RNA and DNA (oligonucleotides). Oligonucleotides are broken down into smaller sugar nitrogenous units called nucleosides. These can be digested by cells since the sugar is divided from the nitrogenous base. This, in turn, leads to the formation of the five types of nitrogenous bases, sugars, and the preliminary substances involved in the synthesis of new RNA and DNA. DNA and RNA have a helix shape.

Macromolecular nucleic acid polymers, such as RNA and DNA, are formed from nucleotides, which are monomeric units joined by phosphodiester bonds. Cells require energy in the form of ATP to synthesize proteins from amino acids and replicate DNA. Nitrogen fixation is used to synthesize nucleotides for DNA and amino acids for proteins. Nitrogen fixation uses the enzyme nitrogenase in the reduction of dinitrogen gas (N_2) to ammonia (NH_3). Nucleic acids store information and energy and are also important catalysts. It is the RNA that catalyzes the transfer of DNA genetic information into protein coded information. ATP is an RNA nucleotide. Nucleotides are used to form the nucleic acids. Nucleotides are made of a five-carbon sugar, such as ribose or deoxyribose, a nitrogenous base, and one or more phosphates. Nucleotides consisting of more than one phosphate can also store energy in their bonds.

Business Calculations/Analysis

TIME VALUE OF MONEY

When money is invested in a safe banking type institution, it can accumulate or accrue interest. The amount of interest earned is called the accrued amount. The interest amount is based on the amount of the investment, the length of time it is invested, and the interest percentage rate. If the money is invested over several time cycles then the interest is calculated differently. At the end of each time cycle the interest is calculated on the increased investment amount which is known as compounded interest. The effective interest rate is the interest rate between compounding cycles. If the effective interest rate is calculated over a year it is known as the effective annual interest rate.

RATE OF RETURN COST ANALYSIS

One of the five common economic comparisons is the **rate of return cost analysis**, simply known as **RoR**. The rate of return analysis looks for the highest interest rate of competing cash flow projection scenarios. A simpler definition is: how much interest would be earned if that amount of money was placed in a bank? Rephrased, that question is also a litmus test for whether a project should be undertaken: would the money have been better off sitting in a bank instead of risked on this venture? This minimum acceptable interest rate is known as the **minimum attractive rate of return (MARR)** and is established by the company. Some companies use different MARR values for different projects or project lengths.

Suppose Rachel has invested $12,000 in restoring an antique car, and $7,000 in Ace Shipping Company. After four years, the antique car sells for $18,000. She sells her shares in Ace Shipping for $9,500 after a year. After calculating the return on investment for both investments and adjusting for time duration, they can be compared.

$$ROI_{car} = \frac{18{,}000 - 12{,}000}{12{,}000} = 0.5$$

$$ROI_{Ace} = \frac{9{,}500 - 7{,}000}{7{,}000} = 0.357$$

Note that to get a more accurate picture of the viability of the investments, the time duration has to be taken into account. To calculate annual ROI, divide ROI by the duration of the investment.

$$Annual\ ROI_{car} = \frac{0.5}{4} = 0.125$$

$$Annual\ ROI_{Ace} = \frac{0.357}{1} = 0.357$$

OPPORTUNITY COST

The opportunity cost of an economic decision is the loss of potential gain from other opportunities when one opportunity is taken.

For example, a person may have enough money for a vacation in Europe, or a new car, but not both. The opportunity cost of buying the car will be the trip to Europe. These decisions are made usually on the utility of each choice - which would provide the most pleasure to the consumer. In a complex economy, there are many competing factors that provide utility. An individual, firm or government will always choose what they perceive to be the best choice given limited resources.

These choices are usually not clear-cut and many factors go into some economic decisions. This is more common when companies or governments must choose between a number of needed and attractive choices. Different parts of society will have different ideas about the best way to use their resources.

NET PRESENT VALUE

Net present value (NPV) is based on the principle that money now is worth more than money later, known as the time value of money. This is because money can be used to make more money, whether that money is supporting a business, invested in the stock market, or put in the bank. NPV is the difference between the present values of cash inflows and the present values of cash outflows. To calculate it, all cash flows must first be converted from future values to present values. This is accomplished by the following equation, where PV is the present value of the money, FV is the future value of the money, i is the decimal interest rate, n is the number of times interest is compounded per year, and t is the number of years:

$$PV = \frac{FV}{\left(1 + \frac{i}{n}\right)^{nt}}$$

where

PV is the present value of the money

FV is the future value of the money
i is the decimal interest rate
n is the number of times interest is compounded per year
t is the number of years

Suppose Ethan's good friend asks to borrow $1,000 from him today, and repay him $1,150 in two years. To determine if it is a good investment, Ethan must first calculate the present value of the sum. Assuming money can be invested elsewhere at a rate of 6% annually, the present value can be calculated:

$$PV = \frac{\$1,150}{\left(1 + \frac{0.06}{1}\right)^{(1\times2)}} = \$1,023.50$$

To calculate the net present value of the investment, take the difference between the cash outflow and cash inflow: −$1,000 + $1,023.50 = $23.50. Thus, assuming his friend can be relied upon to pay him back, it would be a sound investment for Ethan to lend to this friend.

ECONOMIC EFFECTS OF LOSSES

The 'economic effect of losses' refers to the total monetary cost of losses due to workplace injuries. The economic effect is not merely the dollars spent; it also includes the labor cost for employers to manage the loss and lost productivity from an injured worker not being able to perform his or her normal work duties, or performing them at a lower level. Total monetary costs should include the cost of the worker's compensation insurance premium and any employee reimbursements made. Once the total dollar and indirect costs are calculated, it helps to standardize the cost so that different years and plant locations can be compared. For example, costs are commonly standardized according to hours worked. This allows comparison across different years and from different locations.

KEY PERFORMANCE INDICATORS

A Key Performance Indicator (KPI) helps an organization define and measure progress toward its goals. A KPI is a quantifiable measurement that can be used to monitor progress on a specific goal. For example, a company has the goal to "be the most profitable company in the industry". It will have KPIs that measure profit and other fiscal measures. These might include "pre-tax profit" and "shareholder equity", but would not include measures like "percent of profit donated" or "stock price". The main thing to remember is that KPIs must always be measurable, so that progress can be tracked.

BENCHMARKING

Benchmarking compares a performance measurement against a standard of excellence. Companies often seek to compare themselves to the best in class of companies of similar industry and size. In the case of occupational hygiene and safety statistics, the United States Bureau of Labor Statistics publishes data on injury rates by NAICS code; this is a useful tool for benchmarking safety performance. The BLS tracks Total Recordable Cases, Cases with Days Away from Work, and Cases with Restricted Duty. These rates can be used to compare performance in injury and illness prevention and management and are normalized according to total employee hours worked which facilitates fair comparison.

PERCEPTION SURVEYS

Performing an employee survey can be a useful tool to assess the safety culture of an organization. Qualitative data seeks to understand emotions and motivations and is useful in understanding how employees perceive the safety culture. A perception survey can be used to determine whether the safety messages and programs that are in place are understood and followed. It can also determine if a safety program is working. Examples of safety perception questions include:

> *Do you believe upper management cares about safety? Why or why not?*
> *What additional information do you believe you need to safely perform your job?*
> *What do you think is the major cause of safety incidents?*
> *Do you believe the safety rules in place actually protect employees?*
> *What measures should be taken in your workplace to improve safety?*

FOCUS GROUPS

A focus group is a small, informal meeting in which a trained moderator guides the discussion and elicits opinions. In plan making, the moderator is seeking to educate the group on the goals and strategies of existing plans, and to determine their reactions, needs, and concerns regarding development. Group members can be chosen randomly or pulled from a specific demographic population of stakeholders. Although a focus group is not statistically representative of the whole community, they can be helpful in determining how a particular document or plan will be received. To conduct a focus group, planners must abide by these steps:

- *Identify participants.* (They should be pulled from the specific group of stakeholders from which the planners are seeking feedback.)
- Acquire participants.
- *Prepare the room.* (Set up the meeting tables, cameras, etc.)
- Devise questions.
- Find a trained moderator.
- *Conduct the session.* (The moderator must ensure that everyone is involved in the sessions and that no one dominates it.)
- Write down impressions on the session immediately after it is over.
- *Submit a report.* (It should summarize findings, objectives, and methodologies.)

QUANTITATIVE MEASURES TO TRACK AND REPORT PERFORMANCE

Quantitative performance measures provide concrete evidence of actual safety outcomes and the actual effectiveness of safety programs. Quantitative performance measures commonly used in occupational hygiene and safety include the number of: recordable cases, cases with lost time, cases with restricted duty, lost days, and days of restricted duty. Employers track incident rates and dollars spent on worker's compensation premiums. Other quantitative measures that measure actual performance include: number of safety inspections completed on time, number of days required to close corrective action requests, percentage of lifting actions done correctly (this also includes other repetitive actions that have the potential for injury), or PPE compliance.

CALCULATING INCIDENCE RATES

The **total case incident rate (TCIR)** is a health and safety metric that calculates the total number of OSHA recordable injury cases in a year and is weighted by the number of total hours worked by employees at the organization during the year to allow comparison between companies in similar industries. The formula to calculate the TCIR is as follows:

$$\text{TCIR} = \frac{\text{Number of recordable injuries in calendar year} \times 200{,}000}{\text{Total hours worked}}$$

The **days away, restricted duty, or transfer (DART)** is a measure of the number of injury cases that involved days off work, on restricted duty, or transferred to another job. Note that the calculation uses the number of cases, not the total number of days. The calculation is as follows:

$$\text{DART} = \frac{\text{Number of cases with days away, job restriction, or transfer} \times 200{,}000}{\text{Total hours worked}}$$

Ideally, the DART is lower than the TCIR. The 200,000 hours figure refers to the number of hours worked in a year by a company with 100 full-time employees.

Safety, Health, and Environmental Programs & Risk Management

ACCIDENT INVESTIGATIONS

The primary purpose for investigating accidents is to prevent future accidents from happening. Investigations can also identify causes of accidents and injuries, provide evidence for legal claims and lawsuits, and help assess the amount of loss and damage. After an accident, an accident investigation should begin as soon as all emergency steps have been taken to care for the injured parties and to bring the emergency situation under control. Beginning the accident investigation quickly offers several benefits:

- Immediate investigations produce more accurate results because witnesses' memories are fresh and untainted.
- Immediate investigations allow the investigator to study the accident scene itself before it is changed.
- Immediate investigations send a message that the company cares about employees' safety.
- Immediate investigation demonstrates the company's commitment to discovering the cause of the accident and thus preventing future accidents.

Accident investigations should begin as soon as possible. The first tool an accident investigator needs is rope or security tape. Stretching rope or tape around the accident scene will help keep people out of the area, keeping the scene secure, undamaged, and unchanged. Even with rope or tape, though, evidence at accident scenes can dissipate, so the investigator should take photos or a video of the site as soon as possible. Tape measures can be used to mark where items are located and ID tags can be used for marking evidence. Investigators may also need tape recorders to interview witnesses about where they were and what they saw. Particular types of equipment may be needed depending on the type of accident. For example, Geiger counters are needed for radiation releases while colorimeters, sampling equipment, and clean specimen jars are needed for chemical spills.

Accident investigation can be expensive, so it is not always possible to investigate every accident. When determining whether to investigate an accident, managers need to consider the following:

- The cost and severity of the accident. Accidents with high losses, whether in life, injury, or property damage, need to be investigated.
- The frequency of the accident. If similar accidents occur frequently, they need to be investigated.
- Public interest in the accident. If the accident affects the community or is otherwise of special interest to the public, it needs to be investigated to provide factual information and protect the company image.
- The potential losses caused by the accident. If the accident may have large losses in life or property damage, it should be investigated.

PROCESS HAZARD ANALYSIS (PHA)

Process Hazard Analysis (PHA) is an ordered and systematic method for identifying, evaluating, controlling, and responding to various potential hazards in industrial processes. It is a requirement of both EPA Risk Management Program regulations (40 CFR Part 68) and OSHA Process Safety

Management regulations (29 CFR 1910.119). A PHA is required for all processes with significant potential for fire, explosion, or release of toxic chemicals. The specific method for completing a PHA is up to each individual facility but should begin with the most hazardous process first. A good PHA evaluates 'what if' situations, writing regulation checklists, hazard and operability studies, failure mode effects analysis, and fault tree analysis. Any method that considers avenues of process failure and how to prevent and respond to these failures is acceptable. The person doing the PHA must be properly trained and qualified in these methods.

LEADING INDICATORS

A leading indicator is an objective measure that is used to assess actions taken proactively to improve organizational performance. This is a useful measure in evaluating the impact of an occupational hygiene and safety management system because it measures what the organization is doing to prevent injuries and improve effectiveness in a proactive manner instead of reacting to incidents. Examples of leading indicators are: the number of training courses given, the number of safety meetings held, the number of behavioral safety observations completed, the number of area safety inspections completed, and the number of near miss root cause analyses completed. These leading indicators can be used to assess overall proactive performance, and thorough implementation of the leading indicator activities can strengthen the occupational hygiene and safety program.

LAGGING INDICATORS

Lagging indicators in occupational health and safety are those metrics that are gathered after an event—such as a workplace injury—has occurred. They are a useful indicator of the effects of incidents, and they are helpful, but they do not provide a proactive opportunity to prevent such incidents. Examples of lagging indicators are the number of lost workdays, the number of days an employee is on restricted duty, the cost incurred for medical visits, and the number of recordable injuries. While it is essential to track lagging indicators and target improved performance over time, they do not provide a snapshot of future performance. Lagging indicators are often used to assess actual regulatory compliance and are essential for reporting purposes.

INSPECTIONS AND AUDITS

An inspection refers to checking a list of items that are verifiable. It is narrow in scope and is generally implemented to ensure that regulatory requirements are met. Its objective is to ensure a specific task list has been completed at a predefined frequency. Inspections are also conducted by regulatory agencies to determine permit compliance. An audit refers to a review of an entire management system; its objective is to examine a system designed to manage risk. An audit does not generally examine every document associated with a certain topic, but examines a representative sample to obtain objective evidence of conformance.

DEVELOPING AN AUDIT CHECKLIST

The first step in developing an audit checklist is to determine the purpose of the audit. If it is to demonstrate conformance to a third-party certified standard, such as ISO 14001, the standard elements should be considered. In the case of an audit checklist for a management system, a process approach is often beneficial. The audit checklist can be developed for each process to include auditing the elements of the standard relevant to the process. For example, each process will have a training and competence component that should be audited to ensure conformance.

INTERVIEWS

A safety audit can be conducted as part of a compliance audit, a management systems audit, or a combined systems and compliance audit. A compliance audit is focused on meeting OSHA requirements, whereas a management systems audit is concerned with how safety issues are managed according to the "Plan, Do, Check, Act" model. For either type of audit, preparation involves: developing an understanding of the requirements, a list of questions to ask, and records to review. Records to review will include training records, safety inspection records, a review of hazardous exposures present at the facility, how hazards are mitigated, a review of safety communication practices, and a review of safety committee minutes and actions. Interviews should be conducted with employees to gauge their level of safety awareness. Here are some sample questions to ask:

For Employees:
Are you aware of any safety hazards related to your job?
How do you protect yourself from these hazards?
What type of training have you received to safely perform your job?
For Safety Management:
What are the safety objectives of this facility?
How is safety progress measured?
What procedures are in place for LOTO and hazard communication?

PLANNING AND EXECUTION OF AN AUDIT

The first step in planning an audit is to determine the standard that will be used as a criterion for conformance. This will provide the lead auditor with the scope of the auditing needed. Next, the lead auditor should assess personnel resources to determine how to divide the auditing tasks evenly. For many ISO standards, a valuable audit approach is to audit processes rather than individual elements of the standards. For example, training records and employee competence are assessed in the context of a process rather than as an isolated set of records to be examined. The lead auditor should formulate an audit plan that includes the amount of time dedicated to each audit task, who will be the auditor, and who will be audited. Formal notification in advance should be given to those being audited so they can allocate the necessary time and resources. Any audit findings must be presented within the framework of the clause of the standard being audited. A final written report should then be written, with any findings linked to documented corrective actions.

AUDIT FOLLOW-UP

Once an audit has been conducted, proper follow-up is important to ensure corrective actions are completed in a timely manner. Objective evidence is required to verify results. For example, if it was noted that required safety refresher training had not been completed, one would ask to see the training records for the employees at the follow-up. A representative sample of records is acceptable if the total population size is too large to view all of them. For completeness, ask to view the hand-written sign-in sheets from the training class as well as any tests taken by the attendees to verify that the class was actually taken. Other records that are relevant include inspection records, laboratory analytical reports for industrial hygiene surveys, documentation that the chosen hearing protection provides the appropriate level of noise reduction, and examples of training presentations used.

INTERVIEW TECHNIQUES FOR CONDUCTING INVESTIGATIONS AND PROCESS IMPROVEMENT

Proper accident investigation is an important element of root cause analysis. Interviews are best conducted one-on-one because some people are more comfortable discussing sensitive information in that way. The person injured in the accident must be interviewed in a way that is not confrontational or assign blame. Explain that the purpose of the interview is to establish the sequence of events as a learning opportunity and for continuous improvement. Open-ended questions should be asked, such as: "Where were you and what were you doing at the time of the incident?" The interview should seek to establish a timeline of events and to determine what the proximate and contributing causes were of the accident. Questions that can be answered with a simple 'yes' or 'no' should be avoided. Similarly, any witnesses to an accident must be interviewed to corroborate the sequence of events and obtain alternative perspectives.

Process improvement interviews should be conducted with a variety of workers, supervisors, and managers. The interview questions should be open-ended and designed to allow people to freely express their ideas for process improvement. Here are some sample questions:

What steps in this process should be eliminated in your opinion? Why should they be eliminated?
What are some of the inefficiencies evident in this process?
What is the goal of the process?
Are there steps in this procedure that can be combined or rearranged to improve the process?
In your opinion, what are the unnecessary movements of people and/or material? What can be done to remedy this?
How would you improve this process?

CONSULTING WITH MANUFACTURERS, SUPPLIERS, AND SUBJECT MATTER EXPERTS

Manufacturers and suppliers can be valuable sources of safety information. They know best how their products work and which product is best for a given hazard. For example, glove manufacturers should be consulted when selecting gloves for particular hazards. They can provide information on chemical and physical resistance of the gloves and suggest alternative products that may be more cost-effective for your application. When you are purchasing a new piece of equipment, consulting the manufacturer in advance to determine potential safety risks of the process is essential. The manufacturer will often be able to provide safety and training materials. Forklift manufacturers provide training materials for their products and usually have personnel that can come on-site to conduct the training. Consulting with manufacturers of safety equipment such as machine guards can provide valuable information on the right solution for your machine guard hazard. Although consulting manufacturers does not always yield a solution, it is an avenue that should be explored.

There are multiple subject matter experts who can be consulted to promote optimum safe practices. For example, one should always consult the maintenance and engineering staff for input on mechanical and machine hazards. They can provide information on the operation of various machines and the potential hazards, what hazardous chemicals may be used in maintenance activities, and use of emergency shut-off mechanisms. Other subject matter experts to consult are industrial hygienists for advice on exposure limits to determine appropriate levels of respiratory protection. Worker's compensation insurance providers may be able to provide invaluable information to help manage worker's compensation claims to minimize costs while providing proper care for employees injured on the job. In order to minimize ergonomic hazards and prevent injuries from ergonomic stresses it is important to consult an ergonomics expert.

ISO STANDARDS

The International Organization for Standardization (ISO) and Occupational Health and Safety Assessment Series (OHSAS) exist to promote standard safe practices related to environmental, health, safety, and security management. By meeting the voluntary standards of both organizations, companies can achieve various certifications. This gives customers and external organizations reassurance that the systems and procedures in place meet the highest standards. ISO14001 is an environmental management system standard that works on the "Plan, Do, Check, Act" model. It seeks continuous improvement in environmental procedures and performance, and leaves it to each company to design goals, objectives, and measures of progress. OHSAS 18001 is a similar standard that is concerned with employee health and safety programs and performance. It places specific emphasis on employee participation in health and safety topics to ensure a response to employee concerns. ISO27001 is a data security standard that outlines steps companies can take to keep information systems secure. Procedures must be in place to protect computer files and systems from intruders, to protect physical information technology assets, procedures to test the system security, planning for response to information security breaches, and continuous improvement. ISO5001 is an energy management standard. The standard requires assessment of major uses of energy (both in processes and products) and requires implementation of projects that save energy with the goal of conservation and lowering overall carbon footprint.

PROCESSES FOR CONTINUOUS IMPROVEMENT
SIX SIGMA

Six Sigma is a business improvement approach based on techniques developed by Bill Smith at Motorola. It uses statistical tools and project work to identify causes of product defects, and thereby make large gains in quality improvement and profitability. The defect level for Six Sigma is 3.4 defects per million—other possible terms include defects per opportunity (DPO) and defects per million opportunities (DPMO). Six Sigma relies on a disciplined approach known as DMAIC:

- *Define* – Choose the correct responses for improvement
- *Measure* – Gather data to evaluate response variables
- *Analyze* – Discern the underlying causes of defects and nonconformities
- *Improve* – Eradicate the causes of defects or reduce variability
- *Control* – Perform continuous improvement by monitoring processes

If a company wants its workers to learn Six Sigma, it can send them to the Six Sigma Academy. Depending on the amount of training one receives, the trainee can become a black belt (most training), green belt, or yellow belt. The success of Six Sigma lies in its bottom-line focus, manager involvement, disciplined approach (DMAIC), well-defined success measures, short project completion times, solid training infrastructure, and proven statistical approach.

FIVE S

The "Five S" template originated in Japan as a methodology for establishing and maintaining a clean and productive workplace. Is has become known as a lean manufacturing best practice. The five "S" words are sort, set in order, shine, standardize, and sustain. The "sort" is a prompt to begin each shift with an organized work area. The "set in order" prompts the worker to place needed tools and equipment in an order that optimizes the efficiency of the work process. "Shine" encourages continual maintenance of a clean work area. "Standardize" sets forth a goal to standardize techniques, tasks, and processes with visual communication of the standard for workers. "Sustain" is an admonishment to keep the 5S process cycle in place in order to ensure continual effectiveness and safety in the work environment.

OTHER METHODS

There are several methods for continuous process improvement. Lean management improves processes by eliminating waste, which is defined as activities for which your customer will not pay. There are seven wastes to eliminate: transportation, inventory, motion, waiting, overproduction, over-processing, and defects. Lean management uses concentrated multi-functional work groups called 'kaizens' to examine processes and improve them according to established procedures. Product substitution seeks to improve processes by substituting simpler products for more complex ones while maintaining the same quality and outcomes. Sustainability can be thought of as a continuous improvement process, since it is concerned with conserving resources and planning for the entire life cycle of a product. For example, sustainability requires energy, material, and water conservation on a continuous improvement basis. Reducing waste is similar, but is focused on wastes specifically, including hazardous waste, solid waste, and wastewater. Creating less waste and reducing the toxicity of waste in a process is part of continuous improvement. It creates a positive impact on the bottom line by discarding less waste.

BASIC CONCEPTS OF PROCESS SAFETY MANAGEMENT

OSHA's Process Safety Management regulation (29 CFR 1910.119) has several required subparts that must be completed and documented, as follows:

Process hazard analysis: The facility must define an appropriate process hazard analysis (PHA) technique that is suitable for the process at hand and must engage an individual trained in the PHA technique to assist in evaluating all hazardous processes. Examples of appropriate PHA techniques to be used are *what-if*, *failure modes and effects analysis*, and *fault tree analysis*.

Operating procedures: All processes subject to process safety management (PSM) must have written and evaluated operating procedures. These must be communicated to all personnel involved in the process to ensure proper operating procedures in order to prevent fires, explosions, releases, etc.

Training: All employees that work with and around the process must be trained in the operating procedures and the emergency response procedures associated with the process. This training must cover the results of the process hazard analysis and must prepare employees to react to catastrophic failure of the process.

Contractors: All contractors that will work on-site where PSM-applicable processes are conducted must receive training in the process hazards and emergency response procedures. All contractors must adhere to all site-specific safety procedures.

Pre-startup safety reviews: A standard procedure and checklist must be developed. There must also be a formal pre-startup safety review conducted before each PSM-applicable process is restarted after a period of inactivity. The purpose of this is to review that all equipment repairs have been completed, that all systems are returned to the "ready" state, that all employees involved in the process have received the proper training, and that all emergency systems are operational.

Mechanical integrity: A PSM regulation that requires all pressure vessels, tanks, piping, relief valves, emergency shutdown equipment, controls, and pumps to undergo regular inspection and testing according to generally accepted engineering principles or according to manufacturer recommendations.

Hot work permit: A PSM regulation that requires a formal hot work permit be issued for any hot work conducted on a PSM-covered process. This includes any welding or torch cutting. The fire prevention and detection provisions of the hot work permit must be in place before the work is conducted, and the employees must be trained in its use.

Management of change: A PSM regulation that contains specific provisions requiring use of a documented management of change procedure. This requires review and approval of any change to the process by all departments affected by any proposed change, including engineering, maintenance, operations, health and safety, and quality.

Emergency planning and response: A PSM regulation that requires documented planning for emergencies, covering the entire plant's operations. Local officials must be informed of the plan in order to coordinate response. Drills must be conducted to ensure employees are aware of their duties in an emergency situation. The plan must include a response to a release of hazardous chemicals.

HAZARDOUS WASTE MANAGEMENT
CLASSIFICATION

Hazardous wastes are chemical wastes that pose a threat to human health or the environment if mismanaged. Under the US EPA hazardous waste classification system, there are two types of wastes: characteristic and listed. A characteristic waste is any type of waste that exhibits a general characteristic of reactivity, flammability, corrosivity, or toxicity according to established criteria found in 40 CFR Part 261. Characteristic waste codes start with a "D" followed by a three-digit number. "Listed" wastes are hazardous wastes that are either generated in a specific industrial process or contain specific listed chemicals. Listed wastes start with either "F", "K", "P" or "U" followed by a three-digit code. "F" wastes are process wastes from non-specific industries; this list may be found in 40 CFR Part 261.31. "K" wastes are process wastes from specific industries and may be found in 40 CFR Part 261.32. The "P" and "U" lists are wastes that are pure chemical products that are discarded. This list may be found in 40 CFR Part 261.33.

RECORDKEEPING

"Cradle to grave" is a fundamental concept of the federal Resource Conservation and Recovery Act (RCRA). This federal law governs the identification, listing and management of hazardous waste. The law was passed to prevent mismanagement of hazardous wastes that could lead to environmental pollution and harm to human health such as that seen in Love Canal, New York. The Act assumes that the generator of a waste has complete responsibility from the point of generation through to the end of its life (even after disposal). This means that the generator, for example, can be liable for the cost of cleaning up any site they shipped hazardous waste to for treatment, recycling, or disposal. This means that due diligence should be conducted on companies one will ship hazardous waste to in order to determine whether they are managing the waste in accordance with regulations in both the short and long term. One should always retain copies of audit reports, manifests used to track disposition of wastes, and documents on how wastes were classified.

HAZARD COMMUNICATION AND THE GLOBALLY HARMONIZED SYSTEM (GHS)

Hazard communication refers to the Occupational Safety and Health Administration (OSHA) Hazard Communication Standard found in 29 CFR 1910.1200. The Hazard Communication Standard governs the requirements to notify workers of chemical hazards faced at work and to provide information on protection from hazards. GHS refers to an international standard developed by the United Nations to guide hazardous chemical labeling, warning systems, and safety data sheets. The GHS was developed to standardize hazard warning terminology, pictograms, and safety data sheets worldwide so that international commerce could be improved and language barriers overcome. The OSHA Hazard Communication Standard includes the requirements of the GHS. As of 2015, all workplaces in the United States are required to have safety data sheets available on site that conform to the GHS system and to use these in their notification and training programs.

SDS (SAFETY DATA SHEETS)

A **safety data sheet** (SDS)—formerly called a material safety data sheet (MSDS)—provides information on the physical and chemical properties of a substance as well as potential health and environmental concerns. OSHA requires that all chemicals be labeled appropriately and that SDSs be readily available in the workplace. The hazard communication standard also requires that employees are trained, and that the employer maintains records of the training given. The format for an SDS includes sixteen sections. The required sections are as follows:

I: Identification
II: Hazard Identification
III: Composition/Information on Ingredients
IV: First Aid Measures
V: Firefighting Measures
VI: Accidental Release Measures
VII: Handling/Storage Requirements
VIII: Exposure Controls/Personal Protection
IX: Physical/Chemical Properties
X: Stability/Reactivity
XI: Toxicological Information
XII: Ecological Information
XIII: Disposal Considerations
XIV: Transportation Information
XV: Regulatory Information
XVI: Other Information

SDS provide a number of indicators for possible health threats of a particular chemical. They are required to provide all known information regarding carcinogenicity of a substance (known or potential cancer-causing risks). Carcinogenic risks are published in the National Toxicology Program report (NTP), the International Agency for Research on Cancer (IACR), and Occupation Safety and Health Administration (OSHA). Toxicity levels are indicated by numbers called the LD_{50} and the LC_{50}. LD_{50} refers to the dose at which 50% of the test subjects were killed. LC_{50} is the lethal concentration at which 50% of test subjects were killed. Dosages are typically normalized to include the mass of the possible toxin divided by the mass of the test subject. LD_{50} values may also include descriptors that indicate the mode of administration of the dose (intravenously or orally) and the timeframe for death after administration. Limits for exposure to a particular chemical are also provided. These can be measured as the OSHA permissible exposure limit (PEL) and/or the Threshold Limit Values (TLV), which are published by the American Conference of Governmental Industrial Hygienists (ACGIH).

SDS often recommend the usage of chemical protective clothing (CPC). Protective eye goggles with splash guards and air vents should be used when handling chemicals. Face shields should be used when working with large quantities of a substance and are most effective when used in conjunction with safety goggles. If the mode of possible hazard is through contact and/or absorption on skin, appropriate gloves should be worn. Gloves are chosen based upon their permeability to and reactivity with the chemical in use. Personal respiratory equipment may be indicated if fume hoods do not provide adequate ventilation of fumes or airborne particulates. Body protection depends on the level of protection needed and ranges from rubberized aprons to full suits that are evaluated for their permeability and leak protection. Closed-toed protective shoes should always be used when working with chemicals.

REQUIREMENTS FOR LABELS

The term "label" under the GHS of Classification and Labeling of Chemicals refers to the label on the container. Under GHS, it's required to contain certain elements; these requirements apply whether the label is affixed by the manufacturer or whether the chemical is placed into a smaller, secondary container in the workplace. The label must include the identification of the chemical, the manufacturer's name and US contact information, the applicable GHS pictograms, the applicable signal words (either "danger" or "warning," as applicable), and precautionary statements (measures to reduce risk from exposure to the chemical).

PICTOGRAMS

The pictograms used in the GHS system are simple pictures used to convey hazards posed by the chemical. They are meant to be universally understandable by people with diverse language and reading fluencies. They are as follows:

Health Hazard	Flammable	Sensitizer/ Irritant
Gas Under Pressure	Oxidizer	Corrosive
Reactive	Environmental Hazard	Poison

SIGNAL WORDS

Under the GHS hazard communication and safety data sheet system, the term "signal word" is used to describe one word that summarizes the degree of danger posed by the substances. There are only two signal words: "danger" and "warning." The word "danger" is used for more hazardous substances that present immediate hazards such as flammability, reactivity, poison, and so on. The word "warning" is used for lesser hazards such as irritants, environmental hazards, and less toxic substances. The signal word is used on the label to provide a quick and easily understandable indication of the degree of hazard posed by the substance.

BEHAVIORAL-BASED SAFETY

Behavioral-based safety is a system of improving a safety culture and safety performance that concentrates on recognizing and changing employees' unsafe behaviors. Although it is preferable to improve safety by engineering out hazards, it remains a fact that many on-the-job injuries result from individual employees doing unsafe acts, despite policies and procedures that are put in place to ensure a safe workplace. For example, an employee may lift an object without employing safe lifting procedures or may elect to use a tool without donning the appropriate personal protective equipment (PPE). Implementing a behavior-based safety program aims to identify unsafe acts and uses peer observations and corrective actions to improve safety performance and adherence to safe workplace policies.

BEHAVIORAL-BASED SAFETY PROGRAM

KEY ELEMENTS OF SUCCESSFUL IMPLEMENTATION: Behavioral-based safety must first start with a sound assessment of the types of behaviors that are important in a given work environment to reduce the incidence and severity of injuries. Past data on injuries, first aid, and near misses should

85

be evaluated to determine the common unsafe acts that could lead to incidences. These are the behaviors that can be concentrated upon first. Second, teams of safety observers must be recruited for participation in the behavior-based safety program. The line-level workers must be trained in how to make observations of behavior for unsafe acts, and the workers who have performed the unsafe acts need to be notified and corrected on the spot but not in a punitive way. There should also be ongoing feedback to the entire team on the aggregate behavioral observations and how the team is improving over time so that the benefits of the system can be observed.

POTENTIAL PITFALLS: There are potential pitfalls in the execution of a behavioral-based safety program. The successful implementation requires involvement and participation from line-level workers to make the safe behavior observations and to provide feedback to their coworkers. If proper training and support are not provided, the observations made will not be useful. In addition, the team has to understand the potential benefits of improving safety behaviors and cannot be made to feel that they are being blamed for injuries that are out of their control. There should be a definite and observable connection between the safe behaviors observed and the types of injuries and incidents being reduced through improved behavioral performance.

RISK ANALYSIS TECHNIQUES
ROOT CAUSE ANALYSIS (RCA)

Some faults and failures can be dealt with by addressing the immediate, more obvious, cause and effect concerns. RCA seeks to identify the root, or fundamental, cause(s) of the event. The goal of RCA is to gather evidence that can be systematically used to move past temporary fixes to a hazardous event in order to permanently address the fundamental source. As an example, consider a vehicle that consistently overheats. Investigation shows that the vehicle is low on oil. Further investigation reveals that the vehicle is burning oil in the engine, increasing oil consumption. Finally, the root cause is determined to be a damaged piston ring which allows oil to enter the combustion chamber. Replacing the piston ring will stop the overheating problem. Compare this investigation to one that does not find the root cause: putting in more oil or using a better engine coolant may stop the vehicle from overheating for a time, but the problem would likely appear again.

RCA can incorporate a variety of diagrammatic techniques to help evaluate possible root causes. Pareto charts may be developed that focus on the percentage of time a failure was caused by a particular event, allowing the team to prioritize issues to address. FTA can be used to develop a pathway to root causes. Ishikawa (fishbone) diagrams are helpful in the brainstorming process.

GAP ANALYSIS METHODOLOGY

Gap analysis is a tool for determining what steps need to be taken to move from the present situation to an improved future situation. It is performed by identifying the current situation, identifying the goal situation, and then figuring out what actions need to be taken to realize the goal. In the context of workplace safety, perhaps a construction site averages three incidents or injuries per month and has a goal of only one incident per month. The "gap" would be the difference between the current number and the desired one. For the example workplace, perhaps employee training or safety protocols would reduce incident rates.

INSURANCE

Insurance of all types operates on the principle of spreading out risk over a large pool of people or businesses by charging a fee (called a "premium") based upon the likelihood of a loss or claim against the insurance. The insurance company will then cover the cost of the loss, whether it's the cost of replacing a car if lost in an accident or the cost of treating an employee's injury. In worker's compensation insurance, the premium is calculated based on the job classification of the employees covered and the employer's history of work-related injuries compared to other companies in similar businesses. To calculate this last portion, the past three years' history (in terms of number of recordable injuries and total costs) are combined into an experience modifier, or x-mod. Having a better injury record than others in the same SIC code results in an x-mod of less than 1.0 and becomes an economic advantage because the company will pay less for worker's compensation insurance.

DEVELOPING RISK MANAGEMENT PLANS
EXTERNAL THREATS TO CONSIDER

Proper risk management planning procedures must consider all potential risks, the likelihood of each risk, and a plan for mitigating the risks. External risks to be considered include the following:

Natural Disasters – What natural disasters are likely in the area? For example: flooding, earthquakes, tornadoes, hurricanes, etc. What physical and structural measures are in place to mitigate the effects?

Product Malfunction or Contamination – Depending on the business type, an extreme product malfunction or product contamination (in the case of food) is a potential risk. Risk management planning for these types of risks should include a communication plan and a recall plan.

Pandemic flu or other widespread disease outbreak – planning for disease outbreaks should include how workers will be protected, how workers will be notified if the facility must close, and protocols regarding medicine or vaccine distribution to workers.

Labor strike – Although the business itself may not be unionized; it can be affected by labor strikes in related businesses. For example, a strike in the transportation sector can disrupt a business. Proper risk management planning includes being prepared for disruptions in external services such as transportation and shipping.

INTERNAL THREATS TO CONSIDER

A comprehensive risk management plan will include being prepared for events that disrupt production processes, damage the company's reputation, injure employees, or result in a release of hazardous chemicals. Internal risks to be considered in this planning include the following:

Training Lapse – Consider the possibility and likelihood that an employee has not received the proper training, or has not remembered the proper procedure. Management systems should be in place to evaluate whether employees have received the proper training and that they understand how to apply the training in a given situation.

Equipment Failure – Consider what types of equipment can fail that would be catastrophic. Risk management includes developing a relevant preventive maintenance program and stocking relevant spare parts to prevent equipment failures and respond to them if they occur.

Document Loss – Important documents may be lost through failure to implement robust data bank-up and file storage (both on and off-site) and through failure to enforce policies that require employees to store important documents on central servers rather than individual computers. Risk management should consider which documents are essential to the running of the business and to regulatory compliance and take steps to ensure that they are protected from loss.

Hazard Identification and Control

HAZARDOUS MATERIALS MANAGEMENT

HAZARDOUS CHEMICALS

OSHA standard 1910.119 outlines the regulations for the usage, handling, and storage of highly hazardous chemicals. The focus is on preventing the release of chemicals whose chemical properties such as toxicity, flammability, and reactivity have a high potential for disastrous consequences. The regulation requires employers to partner with employees and those with process expertise in developing a system for safe management of the chemicals, including a documented and well-communicated emergency response plan. Appendix A of 1910.119 provides a list of chemicals for which this regulation is mandatory. Common examples include aqueous ammonia solutions that are greater than 44% by weight ammonia, including anhydrous (without water) ammonia. Arsine and boron trifluoride have very low threshold quantity (TQ) limits and are sometimes used in the semiconductor industry. Hydrogen fluoride, hydrogen cyanide, and concentrated hydrogen peroxide are included. Halogen gases (F_2, Cl_2, Br_2, I_2) are all highly reactive and are included in the list of regulated chemicals.

Hazardous waste materials must be handled by an employer-designated HAZMAT team. OSHA recognizes all chemicals listed in CERCLA 101(14) as hazardous chemicals requiring special handling and disposal. CERCLA is the Comprehensive Environmental Response, Compensation, and Liability Act that authorized ATSDR (Agency for Toxic Substances & Disease Registry) and the EPA to develop biannually updated lists of such substances. Examples include arsenic, lead, chloroform, and phenol. OSHA has also embraced all chemicals listed in the DOT 49 CFR 172.101, including those listed in the appendix. OSHA includes biological and/or disease-causing agents as hazardous. Such substances have a high risk of causing death, reproduction interference, or birth defects if released into the environment, regardless of the mode of toxicity.

NFPA HAZARDOUS MATERIALS CLASSIFICATION

The National Fire and Protection Agency (NFPA) has developed a classification diamond that is color coded with a numerical scale that communicates material hazards at a glance. SDS sheets often include the NFPA Hazardous Materials diamond. The diamond provides a vivid "snapshot" of the chemical and is often posted in chemical storage areas. The left diamond is blue and provides warnings of possible health hazards. The top diamond is red and indicates possible fire hazards. The right-hand diamond is yellow and details reactivity hazards. The bottom diamond is white and warns of possible chemical and chemical reactivity hazards.

In the health hazard diamond, a zero indicates normal material, a "1" indicates a slight health hazard, a "2" hazardous material, a "3" warns of extreme danger, and a "4" indicates the material is deadly. In the fire hazard diamond, the numbers specify flash points of the substance, the temperature at which the material could ignite when mixed with air. A zero indicates the substance will not burn. The numbers 1, 2, 3, and 4 indicate flash points above 200 °F, below 200 °F, below 100 °F, and below 73 °F respectively. For reactivity hazards, a zero represents stable material, a "1" warns the material is unstable if heated, a "2" warns of a possible violent chemical reaction, a "3" warns that shock and heat may detonate, and "4" warns of a high risk of detonation. Possible special hazards are **OXY** for oxidizer, **ACID** for acid, **ALK** for alkali (base), **COR** for corrosive, **W** to warn that water should NOT come into contact with the chemical, and the following symbol for radiation hazard:

☢

CONTROL AND STORAGE MEASURES FOR CHEMICALS

Chemicals should be stored separately according to key physical and/or chemical properties. They may be stored alphabetically, but only within a designated group. For example, oxidizing agents should NEVER be stored near organic solvents. Additionally, some chemicals are limited in the amounts that can be stored on-site at any one time. Chemicals must be stored in appropriate containers. For example, some organic solvents will dissolve some types of plastic. Alkaline solutions often etch glass containers. The containers must be appropriately sealed to minimize escape of vapors. Such chemicals are often stored in a cabinet that is vented into the exhaust system. Bottles of chemicals must be scrupulously labeled with the name as provided on the SDS sheet, potential hazards, and the contact information of the manufacturer. Caution signs should be posted at entrances to chemical storage rooms that warn of the particular hazard(s) present. Finally, chemicals must be in a secure location at the proper temperature and pressure needed to ensure stability.

STORAGE AND HANDLING OF FLAMMABLE MATERIALS

Flammable liquids must be stored in approved flammable containers; for example, flammable liquids will generally be supplied in glass bottles or metal drums, not in plastic containers. If a secondary container is to be used (e.g., to transport a small quantity of gasoline), the container must be approved to hold flammable liquids. Flammable liquids must be stored in approved flammable liquid storage cabinets or in segregated rooms that have separate ventilation and whose walls meet fire resistance ratings. Aisles must be maintained at 3 feet in width, and egress routes must be kept clear in areas where flammable liquids are stored.

CONTROL AND STORAGE MEASURES FOR CORROSIVE MATERIALS

Corrosive materials are those that can dissolve metal and severely damage human tissue upon contact. They are usually of either a very high pH (greater than 12) or low pH (less than 2) but can also be other types of chemicals. Because they can dissolve metal, they should be stored in plastic containers. Corrosive materials must be stored away from flammable materials and incompatible metals. Acids and bases should be stored separately from one another due to the risk of exothermic (heat-producing) reactions if they are accidentally mixed. If possible, they should be stored in an enclosed cabinet or room with ventilation that does not go into the work area.

INCOMPATIBILITY

Incompatibility refers to one or more chemicals that when mixed together, create a hazardous reaction. A hazardous reaction can refer to generation of heat (to the point of starting a fire), creation of a hazardous gas (e.g., hydrogen gas, which is flammable), or creation of a toxic gas. Common incompatibilities are strong acids and strong bases (heat and hydrogen gas), ammonia and bleach (toxic fumes), and strong acids with oxidizers. Incompatible chemicals must be stored in well-ventilated areas well apart from one another to ensure they do not mix accidentally.

HAZARDOUS MATERIALS CONTAINMENT

Hazardous materials containment refers to properly containing hazardous materials in the event of an unexpected spill. Considerations should be made when designing containment as follows:

- Containment capacity: What should the containment capacity be? The design criteria are to contain 110 percent of the largest container or 10 percent of the aggregate volume stored. In addition, if the area is subject to storm water, containment capacity must be provided to contain the storm water also.
- Compatibility: Ensure that the materials of construction of the containment device are compatible with the hazardous materials being contained.
- Inspection frequency: Plans should be made to inspect the containment for spilled material on a regular basis. A corrective action process should be put in place to address any deficiencies discovered.
- Emergency planning: What will be the procedure if material is spilled in the containment? Who will be notified, and how will the material be cleaned up?

If the spill is small and the hazards are known, the spill can generally be cleaned up by personnel using appropriate personal protection gear and methods specific to the chemical involved. Exceptions include mercury and radioactive substances. Spills can typically be handled using specifically designed adsorption spill kits or via neutralization. Powdered neutralizers should be applied to the spill from the outside to the inside of the spill in a circular manner. Depending on the chemical, the neutralized material should be placed in a carefully labeled container for appropriate disposal. All sources of ignition must be controlled if the substance is flammable. At least two people should be present in case the person cleaning the spill needs emergency assistance. If large amounts of chemicals have spilled or there is a possibility the spill can result in an uncontrolled release of a hazardous substance, the designated HAZMAT team must be summoned.

HAZARDOUS ENERGY

Hazardous energy is energy that is stored in a machine or device that, if suddenly released, could activate the machine in such a way that it could injure an employee. Stored energy can be of many kinds—mechanical energy (e.g., coiled springs, compressed air) is the most obvious, but energy can also be stored in chemical systems, in steam systems, and as electrical energy. Controlling hazardous energy requires systematic development of a lockout/tagout program that identifies the potential types of stored energy in machines and identifies specifically—for each piece of equipment—how one releases the energy and physically locks the machine so it cannot be reactivated until the service or maintenance is completed and the all-clear signal has been given. Best practice is to post lockout procedures for each piece of equipment at the equipment and to use photos to document lockout points. Ideally, each person has his or her own lock, and each person working on the machine attaches a lock to control the residual hazardous energy.

LOCKOUT/TAGOUT

Lockout/tagout refers to the process of isolating hazardous energy during maintenance activities to prevent employee injury. Lockout refers to physically placing a lock on the power source (to isolate electrical energy) or other means of starting the source of hazardous energy. Tagout refers to placing a tag on the switch to indicate that the energy source is isolated and should not be turned back on without following proper procedures. Tagout systems should not be used unless accompanied by the more robust and undefeatable lockout system, although tagout is a best practice for notifying who has placed the equipment in lockout.

TRAINING REQUIREMENTS

The Occupational Safety and Health Administration (OSHA) lockout/tagout regulation lists specific training requirements for employees both initially and on an annual basis. The training must cover the types of hazardous energy that can/should be controlled (not just electrical energy), what are authorized and affected employees, the specific lockout procedures for equipment they will be locking out, the difference between lockout and tagout, why tagout alone is not an approved control of hazardous energy, and the process to commence safe start-up of equipment after lockout.

AUTHORIZED AND AFFECTED EMPLOYEES

An authorized employee under the lockout/tagout regulations is an employee who has been thoroughly trained in the reasons for lockout and the methods to lock out equipment and has been issued a lock to use. The lock should be personalized by color coding, and/or by the use of personalized tags to notify others who is responsible for a particular lockout. An affected employee is one that has a general awareness of what lockout/tagout is and works near machinery that will be locked out from time to time. However, these employees are not responsible themselves for performing the lockout or for following the steps to safe start-up of equipment after lockout.

HEALTH HAZARDS ASSOCIATED WITH HOT WEATHER WORK

Heat exhaustion and heat prostration are different names for the same illness. They are caused by a victim failing to drink enough water to replace fluids lost to sweat when working in a hot environment. Symptoms include the following: cold, clammy skin; fatigue; nausea; headache; giddiness; and low, concentrated urine output. Treatment requires moving the victim to a cool area for rest and replacing fluids. Heat cramps are muscle cramps during or after work in a hot environment. They occur because of excess body salts lost during sweating. Treatment involves replacing body salts by drinking fluids such as sports drinks. Heat fatigue occurs in people who aren't used to working in a hot environment. Symptoms include reduced performance at tasks requiring vigilance or mental acuity. Victims need time to acclimate to the hot environment and training on ways to work safely in a hot environment.

A heat illness is any illness primarily caused by prolonged exposure to heat. Heat stroke occurs when a person's thermal regulatory system fails. Symptoms include lack of sweating, hot and dry skin, fever, and mental confusion. Victims need to be cooled immediately or loss of consciousness, convulsion, coma, or even death can result. Sunstroke is a type of heat stroke caused by too much sun exposure. Heat hyperpyrexia is a mild form of heat stroke with lesser symptoms. Heat syncope affects individuals who aren't used to a hot environment and who have been standing for a long time. The victim faints because blood flows more to the arms and legs and less to the brain. The victim needs to lie down in a cool area. Heat rash is also called prickly heat. It occurs when sweat glands become plugged, leading to inflammation and prickly blisters on the skin. Treatment can include cold compresses, cool showers, cooling lotion, steroid creams, and ointments containing hydrocortisone. During treatment, victims must keep their skin dry and avoid heat.

CONTROLS FOR REDUCING AND ELIMINATING HEAT STRESS AND THERMAL INJURIES

The keys to reducing heat stress and thermal injuries are stated below:

- Control the source by keeping heat sources away from occupied areas.
- Modify the environment through ventilation, shielding, barriers, and air conditioning.
- Adjust activities by making the work easier, limiting time spent in hot environments, and requiring periodic rest breaks.
- Provide protective equipment such as water-cooled and air-cooled clothing, reflective clothing, protective eyewear, gloves, and insulated materials.

- Incorporate physiological and medical examinations and monitoring to identify high-risk people.
- Develop a training program to help workers acclimatize to hot environments and learn safe work habits.

HEALTH HAZARDS ASSOCIATED WITH COLD WEATHER WORK

Trenchfoot occurs when a person spends an extended time inactive with moist skin, at temperatures that are cold but not freezing. Bloods vessels in the feet and legs constrict, causing numbness, a pale appearance, swelling, and, eventually, pain. Treatment involves soaking the feet in warm water. However, the numbness can last for several weeks even after the feet are warmed. Chilblains are an itching and reddening of the skin caused by exposure to the cold. Fingers, toes, and ears are the most susceptible. Gentle warming and treatment with calamine lotion or witch hazel can lessen chilblains. Itchy red hives can occur in some people when their bodies develop an allergic reaction to the cold. The hives may be accompanied by vomiting, rapid heart rate, and swollen nasal passages. Cold compresses, cool showers, and antihistamines can help relieve the symptoms.

Frostbite and hypothermia are the most dangerous cold hazards. Frostbite occurs when the temperature of body tissue goes below the freezing point. It leads to tissue damage. The amount of damage depends on how deeply the tissue is frozen. Severe frostbite can lead to the victim losing a damaged finger or toe. Frostbitten skin is usually white or gray and the victim may or may not feel pain. To treat frostbite, the damaged body part must be submerged in room-temperature water so it can warm up slowly. Hypothermia occurs when a victim's body temperature drops below normal. Symptoms include shivering, numbness, disorientation, amnesia, and poor judgment. Eventually, unconsciousness, muscular rigidity, heart failure, and even death can result. Warm liquids and moderate movement can help warm a victim who is still conscious. An unconscious victim needs to be wrapped warmly and taken for medical treatment.

CONTROLS FOR REDUCING AND ELIMINATING COLD STRESS AND THERMAL INJURIES

A cold environment can be measured according to the air temperature, humidity, mean radiant temperature of surrounding surfaces, air speed, and core body temperature of people in extremely cold temperatures. The keys to preventing injury from cold environments are as follows:

- Modifying the environment by providing heat sources and using screens or enclosures to reduce wind speed.
- Adjusting activities to minimize time in cold areas and requiring regular breaks in a warm area.
- Providing protective clothing with insulated layers that both wick away moisture and provide a windscreen.
- Providing gloves, hats, wicking socks, and insulated boots to protect vulnerable extremities.
- Allowing employees time to become acclimated to the cold environment.
- Training employees on practices and procedures for staying safe in a cold environment.

HIERARCHY OF CONTROLS

The hierarchy of controls refers to the preferred methods of controlling health and safety hazards. In order of most preferred first, these include the following:

1. Elimination is completely eliminating the hazard through process changes.
2. Substitution is substituting a lesser hazard, for example, changing from an organic solvent parts washer to an aqueous parts washer.

3. Engineering controls are physical modifications to a work station that serve to reduce or eliminate hazards. An example of engineering controls is to install duct work and exhaust ventilation to remove fumes from the breathing zone of the worker.
4. Administrative control refers to worker management as a means of controlling the hazards. An example of administrative controls is job rotation to limit an employee's exposure to repetitive motion.
5. PPE is garments or auxiliary equipment used to protect workers. Examples of PPE include respirators, gloves, Tyvek suits, welding hoods, and steel-toed boots. This is the last item in the hierarchy because PPE is often uncomfortable to wear, and its effectiveness relies on employee compliance, whereas the other methods of hazard elimination do not.

ELIMINATION OF HAZARDS AND SUBSTITUTION TO MITIGATE HAZARDS

Elimination of hazards refers to making process changes that completely eliminate the hazard rather than developing a work-around or protective device. An example would be changing a process to eliminate solvent use. Another example of elimination of hazards would be to change the way parts are delivered to an assembly line that eliminates the need to lifting heavy boxes. Substitution is another mechanism to mitigate hazards. Examples of substitution include substituting chemicals in a process that are of lower toxicity than the original chemical or substituting a tool that requires awkward, forceful grasping with one that uses a more ergonomically favorable grip.

ENGINEERING CONTROLS

Engineering or physical controls to mitigate occupational hazards are changes in the way the process is designed, or the physical controls on the process, that make it unlikely or impossible to be injured by the hazard. Examples of engineering controls include:

- Installing ventilation systems to remove hazardous vapors from the worker's breathing zone, eliminating chemical or hazardous dust exposure
- Installing permanent access platforms with proper guardrails to provide elevated machinery access that will eliminate the hazard of using an aerial lift or ladder to access heights
- Installing a switch on an electrical testing device or press brake that requires two hands to activate, eliminating the possibility of inserting one's hands into the point of operation while it is operational
- Providing machine guarding to protect from pinch points and gears
- Constructing barriers to prevent entry into confined spaces

ADMINISTRATIVE CONTROLS

Work practice controls or administrative controls seek to control risk through policies and procedures rather than physical barriers. Examples of work practice controls are as follows:

- Implementing a policy that any lifting of objects more than fifty pounds requires two people
- Instructing an employee operating a grinder to always wear a face shield during the grinding

Face shields are considered PPE (personal protective equiment); other examples of PPE include respirators, gloves, Tyvek suits, welding hoods, and steel-toed boots. PPE is often uncomfortable to wear. Clearly, work practice controls and PPE are potentially not as effective as the physical controls, as they rely on employees following instructions and policies, whereas physical controls do not present the option to circumvent the control and be exposed to the risk.

SAFETY SYSTEMS AND INTERLOCKS

A safety interlock is a physical mechanism that makes two functions interdependent with the goal of preventing an unsafe condition or act. These commonly involve some type of switch that triggers a machine to turn off under certain circumstances or prevents it from starting up in other instances. It is always preferable to engineer a safety interlock than to rely on employees to follow appropriate procedures. For example, a safety interlock can be installed that prevents a machine from operating if the guard is removed. Other examples of interlocks are vehicles that won't start unless the transmission is in park or a baler ram that retracts if an object is sensed in its path.

The following provides three examples of safety interlocks:

- Kill switches are installed to immediately shut down the associated equipment in the event of a safety emergency. For example, a conveyor fitted with a kill switch will stop moving if the switch is activated.
- On/Off switches in series only allow equipment with many separately controlled switches to be started in series. For example, if a piece of equipment is required to be run with an operational baghouse, the switches can be wired so that one cannot activate the equipment without first turning on the air pollution control devices.
- Switches associated with equipment access ports or doors shut off the equipment with dangerous moving parts if the access door is opened. An example of this type of switch might be installed on a rotating shaft shredder; if the access door is opened while the unit is in operation, the shredder will cease operating to protect worker body parts from getting pulled into the machine.

SAFETY CRITICAL SUPPORT SYSTEMS

Safety critical support systems are mechanisms present in machinery or processes that need to have assured functionality and for which a loss of functionality will result in serious injury or harm, severe damage to the equipment, or severe environmental harm. There are numerous examples in an airplane of systems that must function for the aircraft to stay in the air. Engineers design safety critical systems to be either fail operational (if the system fails, the unit remains operational), fail-safe (if the unit fails it fails in a way that safety is continued), fail secure (which maintains maximum security when the unit fails), and fail passive systems (which continue to operate even when the system fails). To determine whether these systems exist in your environment, ask what happens in different failure scenarios, and consider how emergency non-operation can be taken into account in emergency planning.

INTERLOCKS USED IN ROBOTIC SYSTEMS

Robots are programmable machines used to conduct highly repetitive or hazardous tasks that would be unsafe or much slower if performed by a human worker. Robots are programmed to perform their task. This programming breaks the task into discrete elements that the robot can perform rapidly. Studies have shown that most injuries that involve robots occur when fine tuning the programmed discrete tasks or during maintenance of the machines, as this is when workers are near the robots and an unplanned movement of the robot can result in injury. All robots must have emergency stop buttons; when pushed, this button cuts all power to the robot and it stops moving instantly. Other safeguards are presence limiting devices; in this type of device, if the robot parts or arms move outside of a prescribed area, the power is instantly cut. Fixed barriers can also be installed to prevent other workers from entering the robot's area of motion. Mechanical limiting devices can also be installed to limit the robot's range of motion and prevent them from moving outside a prescribed area. It is also best practice to ensure robotic operations are located away from egress paths, pedestrian walkways, and forklift travel lanes.

HAZARDS AND CONTROLS ASSOCIATED WITH WORKING AROUND PRESSURIZED SYSTEMS

PRESSURIZED STEAM

The most common source of pressurized steam in an industrial environment is created by a boiler system. Boilers are used to generate steam for heating (both process heating and comfort heating), sterilization, food processing, cleaning, humidification, and steam turbines to produce electricity. The use for steam extends beyond the industrial environment to high-rise office and apartment buildings.

There are several safety risks that must be considered when pressurized steam is used in industrial processes. The pipes that carry steam present a burn hazard, so they should either be insulated or there should be barriers erected, so employees do not inadvertently touch the pipes. Signs should be posted warning of the pressure and heat risk. Lockout points should be labeled, and employees should be instructed to bleed lines properly after locking out and before working on them. Fittings and valves should be regularly inspected to ensure that they do not leak or provide a failure point that will allow hot steam to escape into the work area.

COMPRESSED AIR

There are many systems that use compressed air; being aware of them will enable the safety officer to mitigate the risks posed. They are used to inflate tires and other items, power pneumatic tools, provide the air pressure to pneumatically convey materials, and power paint spray guns, sanding equipment, and sandblasting equipment. Air compressor systems must be inspected regularly for leaks, and care must be taken to ensure hoses are free of cracks and damage that may pose a dangerous leak.

Compressed air is a powerful and widely utilized industrial tool, but it poses many hazards that must be controlled. Compressed air produces noise, so noise exposure measurements must be conducted and a hearing conservation program implemented if necessary. Compressed air streams are an eye and skin hazard—if blown directly on the skin or into the eyes, the air can cause serious damage. Eye protection must be worn. Nozzles for compressed air must be Occupational Safety and Health Administration (OSHA)-approved to reduce the nozzle air pressure to below 30 psi. Any gauges used when inflating with compressed air must be tested to ensure they are accurate to minimize the risk of overinflating and causing a blowout.

HIGH-PRESSURE FLUIDS

High-pressure fluids are used in such tools as paint sprayers, fire hoses, and fuel injection devices. Hazards associated with these fluids include air and gas injuries, injection injuries, and whipping of lines. Air and gas injuries occur when pressurized air or gases rupture or injure bodily tissues. Injection injuries occur when a stream of air, gas, or liquid penetrates the skin and enters the body. The fluid can be toxic, or injected gas can cause embolisms. Whipping occurs when fluid moving through a nozzle makes the muzzle and hose whip around. The hose and nozzle can hit people and property, causing injuries and damage. To reduce the hazards of high-pressure fluids, you can lower the pressure level, keep hydraulic lines away from people, use solid lines instead of hoses, and use shields or guarding to separate sprays from people and property. It is also important to train workers using high-pressure fluids in safety procedures they need to follow.

UNIQUE WORKPLACE HAZARDS

COMBUSTIBLE DUST HAZARDS

Dust explosions occur when fine particles of a material disperse in the air and then ignite. The dust can become airborne during a normal working procedure or when dust that has settled in a room is disturbed. Such explosions can occur in a series with an initial explosion disturbing settled dust, causing it to become airborne and ignite. In addition, oxidizing agents in the air can make a dust explosion even more severe. Most organic dusts are combustible in the air, as are some inorganic and metallic dusts. The severity of the explosion depends on numerous factors:

- Type of dust.
- Size of the dust particles (Smaller particles ignite more easily).
- Concentration of particles in the air (Higher concentrations of particles are more flammable).
- Presence of oxygen (More oxygen pressure increases the likelihood of an explosion).
- Presence of impurities (Inert materials mixed in with the dust reduces its combustibility).
- Moisture content (Moisture increases the ignition temperature, making combustion less likely).
- Air turbulence (Combustion occurs more readily and explosions are more severe when air turbulence mixes the dust and air together).

For a combustible dust explosion to occur, five elements need to be in place. Like the 'fire triangle,' the 'combustible dust explosion pentagon' requires fuel, an oxidizer, and an ignition source to occur. In addition to these, a dust explosion must have dispersion and confinement of dust particles. These elements are created when dust particles are suspended in air in an enclosed space. If any of the five elements are not present, a dust explosion cannot occur.

The National Fire Prevention Act standards recommend a variety of methods to reduce the hazards which might lead to dust explosions:

- Processing equipment and ventilation ducts should be sealed against the escape of dust from the cutting, sanding, or blasting activity.
- Dust collection filters and systems should be built into the ventilating system.
- Floors and walls should be smooth and of a type that facilitates easy cleaning. Rough or corrugated surfaces collect and accumulate dust.
- Vacuum cleaners must be specifically designed and approved for dust collection.
- The use of cleaning compounds which collect the dust into heavy absorbent particles on floors is recommended. Cleaning should be done at regular intervals.
- Seek employee input and then develop a written policy for dust containment. Informed workers are a vital part of the plan's success.
- Examine the work area to spot potential ignition systems which can ignite dust concentrations.

SPRAY BOOTHS

Spray booths are enclosures used to spray parts and equipment with chemicals or paint. The hazard posed depends on the type of material being sprayed; however, the most common hazard is exposure to volatile organic compounds or to fine particulates from powder coating. The inhalation hazard can be controlled by proper ventilation, a control device, and by the employee wearing respiratory PPE. The material being sprayed also poses an eye hazard; the employee should wear safety glasses and, in most cases, a face shield. The spray booth itself is considered a confined space if the employee must crawl into it; if it is a walk-in spray booth it is not considered to have limited means of egress and is not considered a confined space. The material sprayed may pose a fire hazard for which an extinguishing system must be available.

DIP TANKS

Dip tanks are vessels filled with potentially hazardous liquids such as acids used for metal plating. Parts to be plated are dipped into the tank. Dip tanks may also be filled with solvents to clean parts. In either case, the dip tank poses a respiratory hazard for which the proper industrial hygiene sampling must be performed and appropriate ventilation provided. It is preferable to control the tank with ventilation rather than provide respiratory protection to employees. OSHA regulations regarding dip tanks may be found in 29 CFR Part 1910.124. It is required that the ventilation control flammable vapors in the work area to less than 25% of the Lower Flammable Limit (LFL); the system must be equipped with a sensor that automatically shuts down the equipment if the LFL exceeds 25%. There must be an emergency shower and eyewash station in the area in case of skin or eye contact with hazardous chemicals. If the dip tank is filled with chromic acid, the exposed employees must be given a periodic examination by a physician of exposed body parts, especially the nostrils.

CONFINED SPACE REQUIREMENTS

A **confined space** is an area with limited entry and exit access that is not designed for regular employee occupancy, but that is routinely entered for maintenance or other activities. The definition includes spaces that even arms are placed into, not just spaces that can accommodate the entire body. Confined spaces are dangerous because they cannot be exited easily in an emergency, they may have oxygen-deficient atmospheres, and there may be dust or vapors present that can pose a hazard to employees entering them. For this reason, OSHA requires assessments and inventories of potential confined spaces to determine appropriate entry procedures.

PERMIT-REQUIRED AND NON-PERMIT-REQUIRED CONFINED SPACES

There is a significant difference between a permit-required and non-permit required confined space. Confined spaces are areas not designed for continuous employee occupancy that have limited means of egress. They may also have the potential for a hazardous atmosphere, either oxygen deficiency, presence of chemical vapors, or extreme temperatures. Entry into a confined space using a permit system is required when there is a potential for oxygen deficiency, explosive atmosphere, and/or chemical vapor exposures. The permit provides a mechanism to track entries and to document that the proper pre-entry procedures have been followed, such as measuring oxygen levels and measuring chemical vapors. Employees must also have an attendant outside the confined space at all times and emergency equipment on hand in case of emergency.

CONFINED SPACE PROGRAM

A confined space program must contain an inventory of all confined spaces at a site, a formal documented assessment of the potential hazards posed by the space (e.g., Is there a danger of oxygen deficiency? Are there potentially hazardous vapors or fumes present? Is there a risk of high or low temperature environment?). A confined space entry permit must be developed and required to be used for all permit-required confined spaces. All confined spaces must be labeled as such, and the label should identify whether the space is permit required or not. The employees that will enter the confined space must receive appropriate training in the entry procedures and what appropriate emergency procedures are.

INDUSTRIAL HYGIENE EQUIPMENT AND EXPERTISE: To fully implement a confined space safety program, one must be able to evaluate whether a hazardous atmosphere exists inside the confined space. The first assessment that must be made is to determine whether there is an oxygen-deficient atmosphere. For this, an oxygen level meter is needed to confirm that the oxygen content of the air inside the confined space is at least 19.5 percent. Second, if there is any possibility that flammable dust or vapors exist, the air must be analyzed for either dust or organic vapors. Organic vapors can be analyzed using a handheld organic vapor analyzer, and the results can be used to establish whether respiratory protection is necessary. The confined space entry plan and testing plan should ideally be overseen by an industrial hygienist to ensure that no potential hazards are overlooked.

CONTROLS FOR WORKING IN CONFINED SPACES

Confined spaces include such work areas as tank cars, boilers, silos, underground tunnels, and railroad boxcars. All these spaces have limited entrances and exits and require specific controls to ensure worker safety. Hazards that workers in confined spaces face include toxicity, potential oxygen deficiency, and fire or explosion from flammable or combustible gases or dust. To protect workers, the following actions should be taken:

- Always evaluate a confined space for hazards before workers enter.
- Ensure that the confined space has adequate ventilation.
- Include equipment for suppressing fires and removing smoke and fumes.
- Train workers on safety procedures they need to follow when working in a confined space.
- Institute a buddy system for confined spaces so two workers are always present.

REGULATIONS DESIGNED TO PREVENT INJURY WHEN WORKERS ARE REQUIRED TO WORK UNDERGROUND

OSHA regulations section 1926.800 describes a variety of directives designed to protect underground workers:

- Entry/exit openings must be strictly controlled and posted with appropriate safety signs.
- Whenever any employee is working underground, a "designated person" must be present above ground. The "designated person" is required to keep a running account of the number of underground workers and to secure and communicate a rescue response when necessary.
- It is the responsibility of the employer to communicate and coordinate with other workers and/or job operations which may impact the safety of underground workers. Movement of heavy equipment is an example of other worksite activity which may impact underground workers.
- OSHA section 1926.800 mandates that rescue plans must be established in the event of emergency. Specific requirements are based on the number of workers employed underground.

OSHA section 1926.800 requires contingency plans for the emergency use of rescue personnel on construction job sites.

- Whenever employees working underground number 25 or more, regulations require that the employer make contingency plans with locally available trained rescue personnel.
- When 25 or more employees are working underground, contingency must be made for two rescue teams. One team must be located within a half-hour traveling distance; the other must be within a two-hour travel time period.
- If less than 25 persons are working underground, contingency plans may involve a single rescue crew which must be positioned within one-half hour travel time from the job site.

Proper contingency planning requires that rescue personnel be made familiar in advance of conditions at the job site.

HAZARDS AND CONTROLS ASSOCIATED WITH WORKING AT HEIGHTS OR ON ELEVATED WORK PLATFORMS

SIX-FOOT REGULATION PERTAINING TO FALL PROTECTION SYSTEMS

Personal fall arrest systems (harnesses, for example), guardrails, and safety net systems must be used whenever workers are employed in construction or walking in work areas six feet or more from the lower level.

OSHA regulations require that the "six-foot" rule be applied to the following situations:

- Workers must be protected from falling through holes or floor openings like skylights or stairwells. Skylights may be covered with solid structural materials. Another method may be to erect a guardrail system around floor openings or skylights.
- Workers employed in framework or reinforcing steel frame construction must be protected by personal arrest systems and/or safety nets.
- Workers who must walk through or work near trenching areas or excavations must be protected by fences, barricades, or guardrail systems if the excavation is six feet or more.

SAFE PRACTICES FOR USING FALL PROTECTION SYSTEMS

For effective fall protection, OSHA recommends that companies adhere to the following practices:

- The company should have a written fall protection plan as part of its overall health and safety plan. The plan should include company rules for how and when to use fall protection equipment.
- The company should follow standard fall protection requirements when fall protection equipment must be used, usually when an employee in a general industry is four feet above the floor, when an employee of a construction company is six feet above the ground, or when an employee is on scaffolding 10 feet above the ground.
- The company should provide correct fall protection equipment and ensure that it is not only used, but is used properly.
- The company should inspect, maintain, repair, and replace fall protection equipment regularly.
- The company should provide supervisors and workers with training on how to recognize fall-related hazards and how and when to use fall protection equipment.

A fall protection system can limit or prevent falls. A fall protection system can include safety belts, safety harnesses, lanyards, hardware, grabbing devices, lifelines, fall arrestors, climbing safety systems, and safety nets. Most of these elements stop a fall that has already started and must meet specific standards. Safety belts are worn around the waist while harnesses fit around the chest and shoulders and occasionally the upper legs. Safety harnesses lessen the number and severity of injuries when they arrest a fall because the force is distributed over a larger part of the body. Lanyards and lifelines connect safety harnesses to an anchoring point while grabbing devices connect lanyards to a lifeline. Lanyards absorb energy, so they reduce the impact load on a person when the fall is arrested.

Personal Fall Arrest System

A personal fall arrest system is a method of stopping an employee from falling from the heights at which he is working. Some personal fall arrest systems involve harnesses, hooks, belts, and loops of rope or other suspension mechanisms designed to catch a falling worker. Fall arrest systems must:

- Not subject an employee to a force greater than 900 pounds if a body belt is used.
- Not subject an employee to a force greater than 1800 pounds if a body harness is used.
- Not allow an employee to fall more than six feet nor come in contact with the floors or objects below.

Personal fall arrest systems must also be able to sustain two times the impact caused by an employee falling six feet. The deceleration distance of travel can be no longer than 3.5 feet.

Types of Fall Protection Systems

When determining what type of fall protection to employ, it is important to consider the task the worker will be performing while using the system. For tasks that do not require much side-to-side moving, a vertical lifeline may be best. If the job includes multiple workers, a horizontal lifeline system may be best. To calculate the clearance required to use a vertical lifeline system, add the lanyard length and maximum elongation distance to the height of the worker's back D-ring. Then add a margin of safety: three feet is common. Suppose a 5'6" worker is attached to a 10' lanyard that has an elongation distance of 3'6". His back D-ring is mounted between his shoulder blades at a height of 4'6". The fall clearance to safely use this lanyard system would be 10' + 3'6" +4'6" + 3' = 21 feet.

Scaffolding

There are many different types of scaffolding designed around specific construction uses. The terminology used to describe scaffolding is varied. Therefore, it behooves the OHST to know both slang terms for the various types as well as the technically correct names provided by the manufacturer.

- Horse Scaffold: This is merely a platform supported on each end by construction "horses" or "saw horses." When made of metal, these are sometimes called trestle scaffolds.
- Chimney Hoist: The technical name for a "chimney hoist" is multi-point adjustable suspension scaffold. This type of scaffold is used to provide access to the inside of large chimneys.

The fabricated frame scaffold is a common type made of tubular steel and welded at the assembly joints. Aside from the mainframe, the fabricated frame scaffold consists of other components like horizontal bearers and intermediate bearing braces or members. Bricklayers' square scaffolding is constructed from a system of framed squares which provide a solid, wide, and stable footing for masons and tenders. A carpenters' bracket scaffold attaches to the building or the stable vertical walls of a building under construction. A catenary scaffold is a standing platform suspended from parallel horizontal ropes or cables attached to beams or other solidly supported structures. Very often, the catenary scaffold is supported by additional vertical hoist and pulley system. A hoist is a manually operated or power-driven device which attaches to a suspension scaffold. It is the mechanism which allows the suspended platform to be pulled up or "hoisted" aloft. There are two common safety devices which are designed to work in conjunction with a hoist to augment worker safety:

- Lifeline: Scaffolds and suspension devices must be anchored to solid structures to prevent swaying, settling, or otherwise collapsing. The lifeline is a rope, chain, or cable that ties a platform to strong and stable anchor points. A lifeline may be positioned vertically or horizontally and fastened at several points.
- Decelerating Devices are mechanisms specifically designed to augment scaffold safety systems. Their chief purpose is to dissipate energy which would harm a falling worker attached by harness or belt. A decelerating device protects against the shock or whip action imparted to a falling body as it strikes the end of a safety line or other implement. It slows and gentles the falling motion.

PRE-JOB SCAFFOLDING INSPECTION

Scaffolding must be inspected after it's erected, before use, and periodically thereafter (daily). Platforms must be at least 18 inches wide and must be secured so that they don't wobble. The scaffold should not block any exits and must be accessible by a ladder or ramp. It should not be erected near any power lines. There must be diagonal cross bracing to support the platforms, and protection must be provided overhead to protect against falling objects. Employees must be required to wear fall protection equipment if they will be working 10 feet or more above the next accessible level.

SAFE WORK PRACTICES WHEN WORKING AT HEIGHTS OR ON ELEVATED WORK PLATFORMS

Elevated work platforms or working at heights pose a fall hazard that can be fatal if an employee falls on his or her head. When using a platform, there should be guardrails that conform to Occupational Safety and Health Administration (OSHA) guardrail guidelines. Employees should be trained in and use fall protection harnesses; the harness must be tied to a place that will safely arrest the fall and not tip over any equipment. If the height is accessible using a ladder, make sure the ladder is on a stable surface and that a coworker is available to hold the ladder and position it so that reaching from the ladder is not necessary. Never stand on the top step of the ladder.

AERIAL LIFTS AND SCISSOR LIFTS

An aerial lift is a basket on an extended arm for lifting workers to heights. A scissor lift accomplishes the same thing but is conveyed upward vertically. Both have guard rails around the platform. Per 29 CFR 1910.67(c)(2)(v), OSHA mandates that workers working from an aerial lift must wear an acceptable personal fall arrest or travel restraint system.

HAZARDS AND CONTROLS FOR LADDERS AND SCAFFOLDS

Common hazards associated with ladders include the following:

- Falling off the ladder.
- Slipping off the ladder rungs.
- The ladder tipping over, the ladder sliding.
- Metal ladders conducting electricity.

To improve safety when using ladders, the following actions should be taken:

- Ensure that ladder rungs are slip-resistant.
- Place ladders far enough from the wall so the arch of the foot can fit on the rung, not just the toe.

- Inspect ladders frequently for damage such as cracks, bends, and other wear.
- Anchor or tie ladders to a support structure.
- Do not use metal ladders around electrical conductors.

Hazards associated with scaffolds include the following:

- Unsecured or loose planks.
- Overloading and structural failure.
- Tipping over, falls.

To improve safety when using scaffolds, the following actions should be taken: Select a scaffold that is rated for the load it will have to support; Inspect scaffolds before use, checking planks, bolts, ropes, outrigger beams, bracing, and clamps; Place the legs of the scaffold on a solid base. Tie the scaffold to a solid structure.

HAZARDS AND CONTROLS ASSOCIATED WITH WALKING AND WORKING SURFACES
POTENTIAL HEALTH CONSEQUENCES

Slips, trips, and falls account for almost 20 percent of all workplace injuries and can even be fatal. Slips, trips, and falls cause strains when the tripping or falling stretches a muscle beyond its normal range or when employees make sudden movements to try to prevent the fall. Slips, trips, and falls can also cause contusions when employees bump their heads, knees, or other body parts during a fall. The most serious slips, trips, and falls involve hitting one's head on a table or concrete floor. Depending on where the head is hit, serious brain damage can occur. For this reason, effective slip, trip, and fall prevention will result in reduction of on-the-job injuries.

SAFETY INSPECTION

Slips, trips, and falls are a major source of lost-time workplace injuries. A focused safety inspection can be conducted to spot problems and correct them before they cause injury. Items to include are cords left across walkways (even walkways infrequently traveled), small objects such as screws, nuts, and bolts on the floor that can cause sprains or slips, spilled material such as oil or water that needs to be cleaned up (correcting the source of the spill to prevent recurrences), rugs that are a trip hazard, uneven walkways or broken concrete, and uneven doorway transitions. You should also examine your workplace to see if there are places that standard work practices require employees to step over conveyors or onto roller conveyors and engineer a solution that eliminates the trip hazard.

OSHA REQUIREMENTS FOR PROVIDING WORKING PLATFORMS AND WORKING SURFACES

OSHA regulations regarding walking and working surfaces require that employers protect employees from slip, trip, and fall hazards and from slippery surfaces. These hazards may exist in elevated work surfaces or walkways, during the use of ladders, when employees are going up and down stairways, when employees have to work on tall equipment, or when employees are working on roofs. These work areas must be assessed and the hazards mitigated through either construction of a physical control (e.g., constructing a platform with compliant guard rails to access elevated equipment rather than using man lifts or requiring fall protection harnesses) or by providing appropriate fall protection plans and personal protective equipment (PPE).

STAIR SAFETY

The following are terms and safety features as related to stair safety:

- Uniformity means that all the steps in a flight of stairs need to have the same dimensions.
- Slip resistance means that the tread on all the steps in a flight of stairs needs to have the same or very similar slip resistance.
- Slope refers to the ratio of riser height to tread depth. The slope needs to be the same for all the steps in a stair. The preferred slop is 30-35 degrees.
- Visibility means having enough light to see steps and using surface finishes that make the steps easy to see.
- Structure refers to the anticipated load the steps are designed to carry. According to OSHA regulations, steps must be able to carry five times the live load and at least 1,000 pounds of a moving, concentrated load.
- Width refers to the width of the staircase itself. Stairs in buildings with fewer than 50 occupants must be at least 36 inches wide. Stairs in larger buildings must be at least 44 inches wide.

EXAMINING THE SAFETY OF LADDERS AND STAIRWELLS

To minimize construction site injury stemming from unsafe use of ladders and stairwells, the OHST must address the following concerns:

- Slippery conditions on stairs and on ladders are a common source of injury. This must be corrected immediately by degreasing or by replacement of ladders and stairs.
- A handrail must be put upon a stairwell higher than 30 inches or one having four or more risers.
- Stairwells and ladders are not storage areas. They should not be encumbered or obstructed with equipment, materials, or suspended objects.
- Ladders must be examined for worn or weak structure. They should be of sufficient length to reach comfortably to the work area. Metal ladders should not be used near electrical power lines. All ladders should be of sufficient strength to support workers and equipment.

HAZARDS AND CONTROLS FOR POWERED VEHICLES

Powered vehicles for materials handling include forklifts, backhoes, bulldozers, etc. Hazards associated with these vehicles include the following:

- Visibility problems because operators cannot always see how well the load is positioned or whether other people or equipment are in the area.
- Falling loads, Overloading.
- Heating and fire from hot engines and exhaust.
- Tipping.

To reduce the dangers from powered equipment:

- Choose vehicles with a rollover protection system (ROPS) such as a rollover bar, cab, or seatbelts.
- Choose vehicles with a falling object protection system (FOPS) to protect operators from falling objects.
- Inspect, maintain, and repair powered equipment regularly.
- Train operators on how to safely use their equipment.
- Ensure good ventilation in areas where exhaust fumes could create a hazard.

- Ensure that pathways are clear of obstructions.
- Use mirrors to improve the operator's visibility.
- Use hand signals to direct the operator when visibility is limited.

FORKLIFTS

FORKLIFT-ATTACHABLE DEVICES

Devices can be purchased that are cages meant for lifting workers to heights using a standard forklift. These must meet specifications with regard to securely fastening to the forks of the forklift, they must be equipped with guard rails of an approved height, the access gate must swing inward instead of outward, and they must undergo regular inspections. Under no circumstances should homemade work platforms be used because they must be engineered for strength and load limits. In addition, OSHA regulations do specify that if one is using such a cage as a man lift, one should obtain a letter from the forklift manufacturer specifying what the load limits are using the cage and that the capacity decal should be changed accordingly [29 CFR 1910.178(a)(4)].

DAILY INSPECTION CHECKLIST ELEMENTS FOR FORKLIFTS

Daily forklift inspections must be conducted by each driver before driving the forklift. Inspection elements include the following: check that horns and alerts are operational; check the parking brake works; check the mast operation for smooth operation and no broken chain links; check the forks for signs of cracks or wear that would weaken the forks; check the tires; check the fluid levels in the forklift, and check for leaks; ensure the seat belt is present and operational; and if there is a propane tank, check for leaks and rust.

FORKLIFT TRAFFIC

A well-designed traffic pattern plan for forklift traffic can greatly increase the safety of the workplace. "Rules of the road" should be established that are enforceable for all forklift drivers and pedestrians. Similar to public roadways, there should be designated lanes of travel for forklifts. Pedestrian walkways should be designated and separate from forklift lanes. Intersections should be posted with a "Stop" sign for forklifts to stop at each intersection. Speed limits should be established and enforced (maximum of eight miles per hour). High traffic areas such as receiving docks should restrict pedestrian access.

PEDESTRIAN SAFETY AROUND POWERED INDUSTRIAL TRUCKS

Although pedestrians always have the right of way, it is important for pedestrians to observe best management practices when walking in areas with forklift traffic. At all intersections, forklifts are instructed to stop and sound their horn; pedestrians should stop at all intersections and look for forklifts. Pedestrians should be aware that forklifts may be backing out of inventory rows. Pedestrians should stop and wait for an acknowledgment to pass through the path of a traveling forklift to ensure that the driver sees them and will stop for them. Never walk under raised forklift forks.

TRAINING REQUIREMENTS FOR OPERATING FORKLIFTS

Occupational Safety and Health Administration (OSHA) regulations governing forklift training requirements are found in 29 CFR 1910.178(l). All employees who will drive a forklift must be trained both in the classroom and on the job and must not be allowed to operate a forklift without direct supervision until they have passed exams to demonstrate proficiency. The classroom training portion should cover the principles of safe forklift operation (the stability triangle), how to determine the load limits of a forklift, how to conduct an inspection of a forklift, how to drive the forklift on ramps, how to carry loads that obstruct the view, and forklift traffic rules. The classroom knowledge should be tested by a written test, and a minimum score for passing the test should be established. Finally, the employee must pass a behind-the-wheel proficiency test to demonstrate skilled and safe operation of the forklift.

LOAD LIMIT OF FORKLIFTS

The forklift generally has two front wheels and one back wheel that pivots around when turning the unit. This three-point triangle formed by the three wheels is the "stability triangle." One must be mindful of the center of gravity in relation to this stability triangle in determining the load limit of the forklift. Manufacturers establish the load limit for various loads relative to the load's center. For example, a 48-inch pallet has a load center of 24 inches. Lifting loads in the air also affects the center of gravity. The load limit therefore depends on three factors: the load center of the object being lifted or transported, the height the load will be lifted, and the counterbalanced weight of the forklift itself.

All forklifts are equipped with a capacity plate affixed by the manufacturer. This plate lists the load limit of the forklift for several common load centers (such as 24 inches and 36 inches). This will be the amount of weight the forklift can safely carry and move, given a certain load center. This load limit assumes that the forklift will be operated at a reasonable speed, especially around corners. Turning corners quickly can quickly shift the load center outside of the stability triangle, causing the forklift to turn over and potentially crushing an employee. Any changes to the forklift that affect the stability triangle or maximum mast height will affect the load limit and the manufacturer must be consulted to determine the new load limit.

BATTERY CHARGING STATIONS

Forklift batteries contain strong acid. Therefore, it is important to observe proper training and precautions when recharging batteries. Battery charging stations should be located outdoors if at all possible. OSHA requires that an eyewash station be available in the battery charging area. Proper PPE must be available to the employee that will be handling the batteries. Gloves must be worn to plug in and unplug the batteries; extra precautions must be taken if a person will be checking the water level in the battery and adding water. Additional PPE to wear when servicing batteries includes acid-resistant gloves, safety glasses, and a face shield. Water should only be added to the batteries after charging and once the battery has a full charge. Only deionized water can be used to fill the batteries. The level should be checked at least once per week, and water should be added to the fill line if it is low. If there is any acid spilled on the outside of the battery, it should be cleaned up using appropriate precautions while wearing proper PPE.

HAZARDS AND CONTROLS ASSOCIATED WITH HAND AND POWER TOOLS
HAND TOOL INSPECTIONS

The term "hand tools" refers to handheld tools that are not powered. This includes screwdrivers, hammers, axes, scissors, box cutters, and pliers. All tools should be inspected before every use to ensure they are in good operational order. One should examine hand tools to ensure the metal is not cracked or thinning to the point that it may break during use. One should also check the handles to ensure they are firmly seated and that any grip coverings are in place and not loose. Tools that are comprised of several parts should be checked to make sure that the parts are securely attached.

POWER TOOL INSPECTIONS

Power tools refer to handheld tools powered by electricity, batteries, compressed air, or internal combustion engines. These tools include power saws, drills, nail guns, grinders, cutting tools, sanders, and riveters. Some inspection elements are common to other handheld tools, such as checking that the metal parts are not cracked or worn and that all parts are firmly seated and not loose. The electrical cord should be inspected to make sure it is not worn or the insulation frayed. The electrical prongs should be inspected to make sure they are not bent or missing (especially the round grounding prong). If there are cutting blades in the tool, they should be inspected to make sure they are not too worn or needing sharpening; dull blades are unsafe due to the extra force required to use them that may cause one's grip to slip.

PNEUMATIC POWER TOOLS

The development of pneumatic hoses to power construction tools is a relatively recent innovation in the construction industry and has presented a new potential for safety problems. OSHA guidelines in 1926.302 recommend:

- Pneumatic power tools should be locked and secured in place to prevent the tool from being forcefully ejected from the power source. Safety clips should be used for this purpose.
- Pneumatic power nailers and fasteners operating at more than 100 psi should have built-in safety mechanisms which prevent triggering unless the muzzle is pressed against the desired surface.
- Compressed air at more than 30 psi. cannot be used for cleaning purposes.
- Pneumatic hoses more than ½ inch inside diameter must be equipped with safety devices which reduce pressure if hose lines are ruptured.

MANAGEMENT SYSTEM TO ENSURE TOOLS ARE INSPECTED REGULARLY

An effective management system to ensure tools are inspected regularly must first identify what types of tools are on hand and in which locations and departments. A schedule of inspection and a responsibility matrix (by job title) must be developed. Finally, the system must include inspection checklists to document findings and follow up corrective actions. Calendar systems can be used to schedule inspections and ensure deficiencies are corrected in a timely fashion. Coupled with routine inspections, random inspections of tools in use on the floor are important as cross-checks to ensure the inspection program is operating properly.

HAZARDS AND CONTROLS ASSOCIATED WITH WORKING AROUND MOVING PARTS AND PINCH POINTS

PINCH POINT

A "pinch point" is a place where a finger or other body part can get caught between moving machinery and a stationary part of the machinery. Although some pinch points are obvious to observers, others aren't apparent unless one closely observes the operation or conducts it oneself. Eliminating pinch points often involves installing machine guarding to shield the pinch point from being accessible to fingers. Some protection from pinch points can also be provided by wearing leather or other heavy-duty gloves, but it is always preferable to install guards.

MACHINE GUARDING REQUIREMENTS

Machine guarding involves examining machines for places or operations that can injure hands or other body parts during normal operation. This includes assessing potential pinch points, rotating shafts that might pull arms or fingers into equipment, exposed chains that might pull hands or digits into machinery, or conveyor belts that may entangle employees. Successful machine guarding involves fabricating guards that shield the employee from contact, whether intentional or inadvertent, from getting caught by or pulled into moving machinery. Entanglement in moving machinery can result in cuts, bruises, and more serious injuries such as amputations. Occupational Safety and Health Administration (OSHA) regulations for general machine safety requirements are found in 29 CFR 1910.212.

MACHINE SAFETY TRAINING PRESENTATION

Training employees in machine safety should include the following elements: presentation of the general types of machines and machine hazards, such as rotating shafts, fan blades, conveyor belts, chain-driven shafts, and sharp edges. This will enable employees to assess new machines and situations for hazards. The methods of guarding against machine hazards include physical guards, mechanisms for keeping hands and body parts out of the point of operation, and safety interlocks such as light curtains and two-hand switches. The employees should be trained in how to inspect their machines to ensure guards are present and the importance of never overriding or removing machine guards.

HOUSEKEEPING

There are many safety hazards associated with poor housekeeping. There is a potential for slips, trips, and falls if there are objects lying on the floor such as boxes, tools, cords, and equipment. Material spilled on the floor also increases the chance of slipping, whether the material is oil, water, or a solid substance. Poor housekeeping and management of oily rags and other flammable materials is a fire hazard if the materials are not properly stored or disposed of. Materials that are precariously stacked overhead are a hazard to employees, who can be struck by falling objects. Improper storage and handling of hazardous materials can result in exposure to harmful organic vapors. Improperly managed containers also pose a spill hazard. Good housekeeping practices contribute to a safe work environment, are more pleasant to work in, increase employee morale, and contribute to increased productivity because employees are able to find objects they need when they need them.

IMPORTANCE FOR A SAFE WORKPLACE

Proper housekeeping and cleanliness are key contributors to a safe workplace. Good housekeeping diminishes slip, trip, and fall hazards by ensuring that tools and work items are put away when not in use. Good housekeeping practices clean up spilled materials promptly, getting them out of the aisles so that employees won't slip on them. Good housekeeping practices help to minimize waste and assist in proper dust control. Proper waste management and storage practices can also minimize fire hazards. Good housekeeping can also help manage tools appropriately and ensure they are not damaged by improper storage practices.

MATERIALS GIVEN SPECIAL CONSIDERATION REGARDING FIRE HAZARDS

Housekeeping is important in controlling fire hazards, especially storage and handling of rags and wipes soaked in flammable materials. If one accumulates rags and wipes soaked with solvents or similar materials, they should be stored in metal canisters rated for flammable rag storage and emptied daily into suitable containers. If rags and wipes soaked with flammable solvents are stored in piles outside of the metal canister, they can build up heat and create conditions favorable to spontaneous combustion. It is also important to store flammable liquids in an orderly manner in cabinets or rooms rated for flammable chemicals.

CONTRIBUTION OF POOR HOUSEKEEPING TO FIRE HAZARDS

Poor housekeeping can increase fire hazards in a number of ways. Poor housekeeping can lead to accumulation of oily or solvent-laden rags and wipes, which are a combustible hazard. Poor housekeeping will also contribute to a higher level of combustible debris lying around, such as boxes, pallets, and packaging material. Poor housekeeping can lead to blocking of paths of egress and exits, which contributes to fire and life safety hazards. In addition, poor housekeeping can lead to accumulation of dust on surfaces and in electrical panels, which can be combustible or cause a short in an electrical panel that leads to a fire.

Requirements for Maintaining Clearance Around Electrical Panels and Fire Extinguishers

Occupational Safety and Health Administration (OSHA) regulations do require that electrical panels have a minimum 30 inches of clearance around them for voltages between 120 to 250 volts. Higher voltage panels require greater clearances (29 CFR 1910.303). In most work areas, lines are painted on the floor to indicate the clearance required as a means of reminding employees not to store materials in these areas. In contrast, there is no specific requirement for a clearance around fire extinguishers; however, OSHA regulations do state that fire extinguishers must remain accessible at all times and that employees must not have to travel more than 75 feet to reach a fire extinguisher if they are working in an area with potentially combustible materials (29 CFR 1910.157).

Hazards and Controls Associated with Hot Work
Welding Project Hazards

There are several hazards to consider when planning a welding project. The safe use of the compressed gases used must be considered. The types of metals to be welded should be considered to determine whether hazardous metal fumes or dusts will be generated that will require respiratory protection (and specialized equipment that will fit under a welding helmet). The eye hazard posed by exposure to the wavelengths of light emitted by the welding process must be considered and the appropriate welding glasses or face shield obtained. The risk of fire and sparks must be considered, and appropriate protective clothing should be worn.

Hot Work Program

Hot work refers to work with hot metal such as brazing, welding, soldering, cutting with a torch, and drilling or grinding that potentially create a fire hazard. Employees engaged in hot work must be trained in the hazards posed by the work and how to mitigate them. A hot work program must include assessment of industrial hygiene hazards (exposure to metal dusts and fumes), assessment of noise hazards, assessment of proper personal protective equipment (PPE; eye protection, proper gloves, and respiratory protection if required) and must include an assessment of fire hazards posed by the hot work.

Hot Work Permit

A hot work permit system is a means of providing a checklist and management tool to ensure safety risks are assessed and addressed prior to conducting a hot work project. The permit should document that the employees have received the required training and have the proper PPE available. The area should be prepared for hot work by scanning the area for flammable materials and moving them out of reach of the hot work. The permit should direct that fire extinguishers of the correct type must be readily available. If a fire watch is necessary, this must be documented. The permit should also document that the required fire watch time period has been conducted and observed.

Supervisor's Duties

Supervisors are responsible for planning the work and ensuring that the hot work permit system is implemented. The use of the hot work permit checklist is a means of ensuring the proper safety precautions are taken and planning is completed prior to the hot work beginning. The supervisor is responsible for ensuring employees have the proper PPE on hand. Supervisors are responsible for providing the proper manpower and personnel to use a designated fire watch employee if necessary. The supervisor is also responsible for ensuring that employees have received the required safety and operational training to conduct the hot work.

SAFETY OPERATIONS ASSOCIATED WITH CRANES AND LIFTING DEVICES

Construction cranes account for a high percentage of workplace injury and accidents on construction sites. The OHST can implement several strategies to minimize injury from unsafe conditions:

PRE-OPERATION INSPECTION

- Before operating, the crane's hydraulic lift controls should be inspected and determined to be in proper working order. The out rigging hydraulic extenders should be solidly placed and fully extended to guarantee utmost stability.
- The weight of intended loads must be within the crane's specified load capacity.
- Human walking traffic should be barricaded from the crane's area of operation. At no time should loads be moved over the heads of workers.
- Cranes must be situated and operated at safe distances from electric power lines or onsite distributive power lines needed for small equipment.
- Rigging and brakes must be examined and trial tested before use. Inspect cable, chains, and hook.

DAILY CRANE INSPECTION

A daily crane inspection program is an essential part of safe crane operation. The presence of appropriate personal protective equipment (PPE) should be confirmed, and it should be checked that access to the area that the crane will be used is controlled. Check the disconnect switch for correct operation, that the hoist is not loose or broken, that the wire rope is seated properly and not twisted or bent, that the push button controls have no damage, that the controls have the required American Nation Standards Institute (ANSI) tag, that the controls operate as they should (e.g., the crane goes up when that button is triggered), that hooks have no cracks or gouges, that the wire ropes are not frayed, and that the capacity plate is present and visible.

MONTHLY CRANE INSPECTION

There are additional inspection elements for a monthly crane inspection above the daily requirements. All inspections must be conducted by qualified personnel. Items to be inspected include looking for deformed, cracked, or corroded members; loose bolts and rivets; cracked or worn sheaves and drums; worn bearings, pins, shafts, or gears; and excessive wear on brake system and parts. Check that the load indicators function correctly over the full operating range, and check for excessive wear on chain drive sprockets.

CRANE LOAD RATINGS

Manufacturers of cranes design them for a certain load capacity. The load capacity is the maximum that the crane can safely lift; however, it is not good practice to lift approaching the capacity limit unless the crane is designed for that type of use. Cranes are classified as follows:

- Class A: Standby service—crane on standby or used infrequently
- Class B Light service—used at slow speeds and infrequently
- Class C Moderate service—Average 50 percent of rated capacity, five to ten lifts per hour
- Class D Heavy service—Used at 50 percent of rated capacity constantly through the work day
- Class E Severe service—Used approaching capacity 20 times per hour
- Class F Continuous severe service—Used approaching capacity continuously throughout its life

CHAIN FALL

A chain fall is a type of hoist that uses a chain that loops over a pulley to lift heavy objects. Many are equipped with electronic controls and are powered to move the object being lifted. The hazards of using a chain fall occur if the load becomes unbalanced, if the chain fall doesn't stop when powered off, and if the wire rope or chain breaks during the lift. Employees can be struck or crushed by heavy objects. Safe use includes proper employee training, the use of PPE, and completing a pre-use inspection. Inspection elements include ensuring all controls work as intended, the unit stops when powered off, the hook and hook latch are not damaged, the wire rope or chain is not notched or frayed, there are no oil leaks in the unit, and the safety warning signs are intact. The area around the unit and work area should be inspected to ensure there are no obstacles or trip hazards that would interfere with movement of employees or materials during use of the chain fall.

SAFETY PROCEDURES ASSOCIATED WITH RIGGING AND HOISTING
PRE-JOB INSPECTION OF RIGGING EQUIPMENT

A pre-job safety inspection must be conducted before any rigging job. Ensure all lines to be used are not frayed or broken. Ensure all employees are aware of how the job is planned to be conducted and are aware of their respective roles. Ensure the controls on the equipment operate as planned and that the equipment is parked in a stable surface and will not rock once the load is engaged and lifted. Inspect hydraulic lines for leaks, and ensure there are proper levels of hydraulic fluid. Evaluate the need for tag lines, and employ them if necessary.

TAG LINES

Tag lines are used in the use of cranes and hoisting equipment to attach to and stabilize the object being lifted. Lifting and moving an object with a crane will cause the load to swing on the end of the cable like a pendulum, which is potentially dangerous to employees. The tag lines are affixed to the load and to the ground to stabilize the load and prevent it from swinging. The tag lines must be made of soft material such as nylon or sisal, not of wire rope. Tag lines are required when the risk to employees of being hit by a swinging load exists or when there are overhead electrical lines that may be hit by a swinging load or crane.

WIRE ROPE USED IN CONSTRUCTION RIGGING

The use of wire rope for construction rigging must meet OSHA specifications:

- There cannot be more than three full tucks in a wire rope. Other permitted types of connection may be used if they meet safety specifications.
- Wire ropes used for hoisting or lowering must be constructed of a continuous length of rope without knot or splice except for the eye splices at the end of the rope.
- The eyes in wire rope slings or bridles must not be comprised of wire rope clips or knots.
- Wire rope shouldn't be used if the total number of visible broken wires is in excess of ten percent of the total number of wires. Nor can wire rope be used if the rope shows other signs of excessive corrosion or wear.
- Store rigging properly, out of sunlight and away from moisture and chemicals that can cause it to deteriorate.
- Inspect rigging regularly to ensure it is not deteriorating or wearing out.
- Follow load capacity charts for rigging to guard against overloading.

HAND SIGNALS FOR COMMUNICATING IN A RIGGING AND HOISTING JOB

Hand signals should be used whenever the crane operator cannot see the load or landing area or cannot see the path of travel or when the load is close to power lines. Signals should be communicated bare-handed. The common signals are as follows:

- HOIST—Raise the arm at the elbow with the index finger pointing up, then move hand in a horizontal circle.
- LOWER—Lower the arm straight down with the index finger down, then move the hand in a horizontal circle, pointing down.
- BOOM UP—Extend right arm to the side with fingers closed and thumb pointing up.
- BOOM DOWN— Extend right arm to the side with fingers closed and thumb pointing down.
- TRAVEL FORWARD—With palm up, move the thumb in the direction of travel.
- STOP—Extend the arm straight out with palm down.
- EMERGENCY STOP—With the arm extended straight out, palm down, move rapidly right and left.

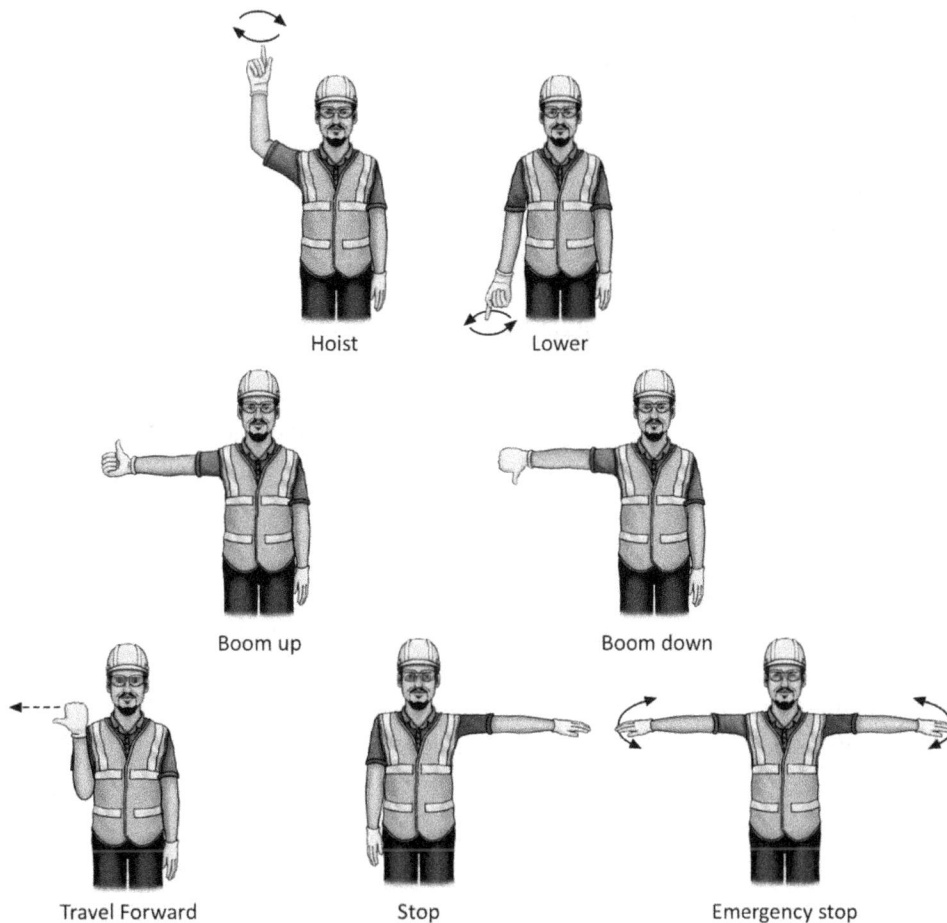

Hoist   Lower

Boom up   Boom down

Travel Forward   Stop   Emergency stop

PERSONAL PROTECTIVE EQUIPMENT (PPE)

Personal protective equipment is any specialized clothing or equipment worn or used to protect a person from hazards. Personal protective equipment can include HAZMAT suits, goggles, gloves, respiration equipment, hard hats, and more. Personal protective equipment can form an essential part of a safety plan, but it should never be a primary means for controlling hazards. Personal

111

protective equipment forms a barrier between the user and a hazard, but it does not remove the hazard. It is far better to remove the hazard, if possible. Personal protective equipment has limited success because the user must have the right equipment and know how to use it properly, often in an emergency situation. In addition, the personal protective equipment must fit properly and must be well-maintained.

In order to be effective, a program for personal protective equipment must include detailed, written procedures that address how to select, manage, use, and maintain personal protective equipment. These procedures must be enforced and supported by management and should include standards and rules for the following:

- Wearing and using personal protective equipment.
- Inspecting and testing personal protective equipment to ensure it is in good condition and working properly.
- Maintaining, repairing, cleaning, and replacing personal protective equipment.

Another important element of a personal protective program is to ensure that users understand and accept the importance of personal protective equipment. Allowing users to participate in selecting the personal protective equipment they will wear can help them "buy into" the program and be more likely to use their personal protective equipment when it is needed.

EYES AND EARS

Eyes need to be protected from flying particles and objects, splashing liquids, excessive light, and radiation. Types of eye protection include spectacles, with or without side shields, and goggles. Spectacles and goggles protect the eyes from frontal impact injuries, particles, splashes, etc. Side shields are needed for spectacles if there is any danger of particles hitting the eyes from the side. Spectacle lenses can be tinted to prevent light damage and include radiation filters. Different types of spectacles and goggles are available for different tasks. For example, employees working with lasers need laser safety goggles that can filter the specific wavelength and intensity of the laser beam. Hearing needs to be protected from excessive noise, or hearing loss can result. Two main types of hearing protection are muffs and earplugs. Muffs are best for very noisy environments. For the noisiest environments, muffs and plugs can be used together.

HEAD AND FACE

Personal protective equipment for the head can protect wearers from being hit by falling or flying objects, from bumping their heads, and from having their hair caught in a machine or set on fire. Helmets bump caps, and hard hats are examples of this type of head protection. Hoods and soft caps are another type of head protection that also protects the face and neck. Hoods may include hardhat sections as well as air supply lines, visors, and other protective features. They provide protection from heat, sparks, flames, chemicals, molten metals, dust, and chemicals. Head protection can also aid sanitation by keeping hair and skin particles from contaminating the work. This is especially important in processes involving food and clean room work. Hairnets and caps offer this type of protection. Face shields and welding helmets protect the face from sparks, molten metal, and liquid splashes. They should always be used in conjunction with eye protection such as goggles or spectacles.

HANDS, FINGERS, ARMS, FEET, AND LEGS

Hands, feet, arms, fingers, and legs need protection from heat and cold, sharp objects, falling objects, chemicals, radiation, and electricity. Gloves and mittens protect the hands and fingers and can even extend up the wrist and arm. They can be made of different materials according to the protection needed: for example, lead is used for radiation protection and leather for protection from sparks. Gloves can be fingerless to protect just the hands; finger guards are used to protect just the fingers. Creams and lotions also protect hands and fingers from water, solvents, and irritants. Feet can be protected by the appropriate type of shoes: safety shoes with steel toes and insoles; metatarsal or instep guards; insulated shoes; and slip-resistant, conductive, or non-conductive soles. Rubber or plastic boots provide protection against water, mud, and chemicals while non-sparking and non-conductive shoes are useful for people working around electricity or where there is a danger of explosion. Shin guards and leggings protect legs from falling and moving objects and from cuts from saws and other equipment.

RESPIRATORY PROTECTION

Respiratory protection can mean ensuring that air for breathing is of good quality or it can mean cleaning air before it is inhaled. Two types of equipment ensure that air is of good quality: self-contained respirators and supplied-air respirators. Air-purifying respirators clean air before it is inhaled. Self-contained breathing apparatuses (SCBA) are an example of a self-contained respirator. SCBAs are usually enclosed in a backpack and provide users with clean, breathable air. Hose masks, air-line respirators, and air-supplied suits and hoods are all examples of supplied-air respirators. These units provide breathable air to the wearer through a hose from an outside source. Air-purifying respirators use filters, cartridges, or canisters to remove particulates and gases from air. Different types of filters, cartridges and canisters are available for different types of contaminants.

BODY PROTECTION

Personal protective equipment for the body provides protection from hazardous materials, biohazards, heat, fire, sparks, molten metal, and dangerous liquids. This clothing is often combined with other types of personal protective equipment, such as respiratory equipment and eye protection. Types of personal protective equipment for the body include the following:

- Coats and smocks to protect clothing from spills
- Coveralls, which may include hoods and boots
- Aprons, which protect the front of a person from spills and splatters
- Full body suits for working with substances that present a danger to life or health (may include cooling units to help lower the wearer's body temperature)
- Fire entry suits
- Rainwear
- High-visibility clothing for people working on road construction or in traffic
- Personal flotation devices for people working around or on water
- Puncture-resistant or cut-resistant clothing for protection from ballistic objects, power saws and other cutting equipment

Some personal protective equipment is designed to be disposable, especially clothing contaminated with hazardous materials.

STORAGE AND MAINTENANCE

Proper storage and maintenance of personal protective equipment is important for personal hygiene and for proper operation of the equipment. The following covers storage and maintenance procedures for respirators, hearing protection, and gloves:

Respirators – Respirators must be stored in a sealed plastic bag to protect them from being contaminated by dust. Best practice dictates that respirators are only stored after they are thoroughly cleaned and dry. Maintenance of respirators requires that all inhalation and exhalation valve flaps be in place and replaced if worn, and that filter cartridges be replaced according to a pre-established schedule or whenever breakthrough is detected.

Hearing Protection – Ear plug hearing protection should only be inserted using clean hands. If ear plugs are soiled or fall on the ground, they should be replaced. They should be stored in a plastic bag away from potential dust contamination. Replacement of disposable earplugs should be done weekly if they are worn daily, or if they seem to be losing elasticity. Ear muff hearing protection needs only to be cleaned off periodically. They should be replaced if they are cracked or worn and do not provide a good seal around the ears.

Gloves – should be stored in a locker or other area away from dust. They must be examined before each use to ensure there are no holes or tears. Gloves should be replaced when worn out.

INSPECTION

Once the proper personal protective equipment is selected in accord with a job hazard analysis, it must be properly inspected and maintained. Whenever possible, employees should be assigned their own PPE devices and should not have to share with another employee. Certain types of PPE must be inspected for proper configuration before each use, such as fall protection equipment and respirators. High-value and high-risk PPE should be inventoried and documented inspections conducted (for example, fall protection equipment and SCBA respirators). Assigning the equipment to a particular person is essential so that any deviations from inspection procedures or misplaced equipment can be identified and the offending employee counseled. All PPE used for emergency purposes must be inspected at least monthly, and these inspections should be documented to show they have been conducted.

ELECTRICAL SAFE WORK PRACTICES

Electricity is dangerous due to the potential for shock and electrical burns. Basic electrical safety for non-electricians includes the following: never use tools or equipment with worn or frayed wiring or that do not have the wire insulation intact, never use cords with damaged prongs or if the ground (round) prong is missing, do not use electricity around water (water is a good conductor of electricity and amplifies the risk), do not enter electrical panels, especially if they are high voltage, always be aware of the voltage you are working with, be familiar with basic first aid for victims of electrical shock, and never attempt repairs if you are not trained and qualified for electrical work.

The Occupational Safety and Health Administration (OSHA) Electrical Safety Standard (29 CFR 1910.303) considers that guarding and personal protective equipment (electrical safety gloves or other measures) must be taken when employees are exposed to live electrical wires greater than 50 volts. Many companies have adopted more stringent requirements that require protection if exposure levels are greater than 30 volts. Electrical safety gloves must be worn, and untrained and unauthorized employees must stay at least 10 feet from the energized parts. There must be a means of triggering an emergency stop available to the employee, and there must be personnel on site who are trained in first aid measures for electric shock if employees will be exposed to electricity above these threshold levels.

ARC FLASH

Arc flash is an event in which electrical current jumps (or flows) through an air gap between two conductors; for example, broken or torn wire insulation can cause conditions that promote arc flash, as can dust buildup in an electrical panel. Arc flash is an extremely dangerous condition due to the tremendous energy released during the event. The arc flash explosion can cause severe burns, and the explosive concussion can throw an employee some distance from the event. It can also cause hearing damage. Unfortunately, the susceptibility of a given electrical panel to arc flash is not apparent to the naked eye, making an arc flash assessment and electrical panel labeling program important.

SAFETY PROGRAM

All electrical workers must be trained in the basic elements of arc flash safety. All electrical panels must be evaluated by qualified personnel to determine the arc flash potential. This evaluation considers the potential release of energy that would occur (based on voltage and load) were there to be an arc flash in that panel. From this, the panel is rated on a scale of 0 to 4. Personnel that will be working in the panel must wear personal protection suits rated for the appropriate arc flash hazard level. In addition, workers must be trained to set up appropriate exclusion zones around areas where work will occur on electrical panels. Workers must be trained in emergency procedures and first aid procedures for victims of electrical shock and burns.

TEMPORARY POWER CORD SAFETY

Temporary power cords and extension cords should only be used on a short-term basis. They should not be installed as substitutes for permanent wiring. Any actual wiring work must be performed by a qualified electrical worker that has been trained under OSHA requirements and NFPA 70E. Extension cords should always be examined before use to ensure they are not frayed or the insulation missing and that the third ground prong is in place and not bent. Care must be taken to install the cords in such a way that they do not pose a trip hazard; for example, use a cord protector do not trip over it. If the cord will be used for electronic equipment or computers, it should have a surge protector in it to protect the electronic equipment against power surges.

GFCI

A Ground Fault Circuit Interrupter (GFCI) protects against the most common type of electrical shock, a ground fault. A ground fault occurs when an electrical current finds an alternate 'path of least resistance' to the ground (or earth) than the ground wire. A person receives a shock when this path of least resistance is through their body. GFCIs are commonly used and required in wet areas such as bathrooms or kitchens, since the presence of water increases the chance that electrical current will experience a ground fault. Water is very conductive and provides an easy path for electrical current. The GFCI works by comparing the current that exits the unit to the current returning to it; if a significant difference is detected, it immediately cuts off the electricity flow through the circuit and protects from the risk of electrical shock.

HAZARDS AND CONTROLS ASSOCIATED WITH EXCAVATIONS
TRAINING REQUIREMENTS

As part of a comprehensive injury prevention plan and hazard communication plan, workers who work in an excavation site must be trained on the hazards of an excavation and how they are protected from injury. They should be trained in site-specific emergency procedures. If wearing a harness, the employee must be trained in how to use the harness and how to inspect it to ensure it is working optimally.

SAFETY CONSIDERATIONS WHEN PLANNING PROJECTS

A trenching or excavation project poses many safety hazards that must be carefully considered through a site-specific pre-job planning process; potential cave-ins are the greatest risk. Considerations must be given to the type of soil to be excavated, and cave-in prevention measures will be taken according to the type of soil, location of underground and overhead utility lines, the weather forecast, and the potential for a hazardous atmosphere in the trench or excavation. Consideration must be made for the types of personal protective equipment (PPE) the employees

115

will need. Everyone should wear a high-visibility vest, and if entering excavations of a deep and confined space, employees must wear a harness and lifeline. Provisions should be made for daily inspections for excavation integrity; inspections should also be done when conditions have changed in the excavation (e.g., due to weather).

SOIL TYPES

The type of soil to be excavated into is important in determining the proper safety measures that must be taken. A qualified soil classification specialist must perform the determination and make the recommendations. The **unconfined compressive strength** is the load at which the soil will fail; it must be evaluated, either in the field or in the laboratory. The basic soil types are as follows:

- Stable rock: This is natural solid material that can be excavated and remain intact while work is performed in the excavation.
- Type A soil: This is soil that has an unconfined compressive strength of 1.5 tons per square foot or greater. These soils are described as clay, silty clay, sandy clay, or clay loam.
- Type B soil: This is soil that has an unconfined compressive strength of 0.5 to 1.5 tons per square foot. It may be described as crushed rock, angular gravel, silt loam, or sandy loam.
- Type C soil: This is soil that has an unconfined compressive strength of less than 0.5 tons per square foot. This type of soil may have water seeping from it or may be a layered system that reaches into the trench or excavation.

SAFETY REQUIREMENTS

The risk of a cave-in is the greatest risk at an excavation site. Any excavation of greater than five feet deep must have a protective system in place to prevent cave-ins (barricades, sloping side, benching, etc.). If the excavation is greater than twenty feet deep, this protective system must be designed by a registered professional engineer. There are several types of cave-in protection available, such as shoring the sides, sloping the sides to reduce the vertical edge, benching the sides, and shielding workers from the sides. A qualified individual should be consulted when choosing cave-in protection, as site conditions such as soil type, moisture level, and the amount of activity around the excavation must be taken into consideration. Access and egress to the excavation area and the excavation itself must be controlled with barricades and work practice controls. A ladder or ramp must be provided as a means of egress if the depth of the excavation is four feet or greater. The route to the means of egress cannot be more than 25 feet for any employee who may be working in the excavation. The spoil pile (the soil removed from the pit) must be set back from the edge of the excavation at least two feet. This prevents material falling on workers and makes an even walking surface at the edge of the excavation.

CONDUCTING THE REQUIRED DAILY INSPECTION OF AN ONGOING EXCAVATION SITE

Daily inspections of excavation sites are required as a minimum but inspections can be made at any time a change in work, weather, or environmental conditions makes more frequent inspections desirable. The safety inspector must be alert to all hazardous conditions affecting worker safety but there are certain commonalities of concern:

- Examine for failure of protective systems, hazardous atmospheres, water accumulation and the ground signs which may indicate a potential collapse of excavation walls.
- Means of exit or egress should be inspected. Stairways, ladders, ramps or other safe means of evacuation from trenches are required in ditches or trenches that are 4 feet or more in depth. A worker should not have to travel more than 25 feet to reach a means of safe exit.
- Stability of adjoining walls, buildings, or other nearby structures should be inspected for settling, leaning, or other signs of tipping.

SAFETY PRACTICES ASSOCIATED WITH MOTOR VEHICLE OPERATION
LOADING DOCK SAFETY PROGRAM
An effective dock safety program involves controlling driver behavior, dock employee behavior, and putting in place physical controls. All employees working in the dock area should wear high-visibility vests (including visitors). All trucks and trailers parked in the dock should be required to use wheel chocks. A stoplight signal system should be installed to indicate green when the truck or trailer can be removed from the dock. Trailers parked in the dock with no truck tractor attached should be supported by a trailer jack. Any physical controls (such as the stoplight system and use of chocks) should be inspected monthly to ensure they are operational and that employees are using them.

SAFETY TRAINING TO OPERATE MOTOR VEHICLES
Employees who will operate motor vehicles during work hours, whether their own or company vehicles, should receive a basic driver safety class. Driving license or credentials should be verified to ensure the person is a licensed driver. Prohibitions on driving while under the influence of alcohol or drugs should be made explicit. Drivers should also be educated about the dangers of texting or e-mailing while driving, and company policy should prohibit this. Employers should also consider disallowing phone calls while driving, even with a hands-free device, as studies have shown even talking on the phone decreases attention. Employees should be educated on defensive driving techniques and how to respond when there is an accident (who to notify in the company and how to notify the police).

SCREENING OF EMPLOYEES WHO WILL OPERATE NONCOMMERCIAL COMPANY VEHICLES
When employees will operate motor vehicles during work time or for work purposes, the employer should do basic screening, even if the employee will be driving his or her own vehicle. This is because any accidents that happen during the course of work activities are considered work related and will incur employer insurance liability. Employers should check to ensure that drivers are properly licensed and carry appropriate automobile liability insurance. It may be appropriate to require that employees enroll in their state's pull notice program (this service automatically notifies the employer if the driver has any accidents, citations for driving under the influence, or tickets).

SCREENING OF EMPLOYEES WHO WILL OPERATE A COMMERCIAL COMPANY VEHICLE
Operating a commercial company vehicle is a big responsibility. The employee must have his or her driving credentials checked to ensure he or she holds the proper license for the vehicle he or she will drive (Class A, B, or C). Employees who will transport hazardous waste or hazardous materials must have a hazardous endorsement on their license. If they will be covered under the US Department of Transportation (DOT) rules, they must have a DOT physical exam and a DOT drug and alcohol screen prior to starting employment. Employees who will operate company commercial vehicles should also have a driver proficiency test given by another experienced employee to demonstrate they can actually drive the vehicles they are licensed to drive.

STANDARD PROCEDURES FOR FORKLIFT ENTRY INTO A TRUCK TRAILER
Failure to follow safe entry procedures before entering a truck trailer with a forklift can prove fatal. Ensure the truck brake is on and the wheels are chocked. Make sure the trailer can bear the weight of the forklift and that the mast height of the forklift will not bump the roof of the trailer. Make sure the dock signal light (if any) shows that the truck side is red and the dock side is green. Inspect the floor of the trailer for debris, and remove it prior to entry. Ensure the dock plate is secure and

provides a level entry surface to enter the trailer. Always drive forklifts forward into the trailer and reverse out of the trailer.

DEFENSIVE DRIVING TECHNIQUES

Defensive driving refers to a process of alert driving behavior that attempts to anticipate road hazards and actions of other drivers in such a way as to prevent accidents. A key part of defensive driving is paying attention to road conditions and other drivers' behaviors. For example, when changing lanes, drivers should not move into a lane that has a vehicle directly opposite in another lane that can also move into the lane at the same time; this avoids a potential sideswipe collision. Other examples of defensive driving include not following vehicles too closely, staying at or near the speed limit, allowing plenty of time to stop a vehicle, and reducing speed when being passed by another vehicle. Defensive drivers yield when there is a potential collision and follow all posted signs.

SAFETY PRACTICES ASSOCIATED WITH HEAVY EQUIPMENT OPERATION

SAFETY EQUIPMENT

Heavy equipment must be equipped with safety features before use. All vehicles must have seatbelts for the operator to wear. All heavy equipment vehicles must have a service brake system, an emergency brake, and a parking brake. The equipment must be equipped with an audible warning device (horn), headlights, taillights, and brake lights. The unit must also have an intact windshield and windshield wipers. It is a good idea to have a fire extinguisher on hand and a system for emergency communication with the driver (such as radio or cell phone).

HIGHEST SAFETY RISKS

Heavy equipment operation carries with it risks of rollover and of hitting bystanders. These risks are mitigated by making sure the equipment is inspected before each use and is equipped with safety features such as rollover protection devices (a cage for the operator and safety restraints) and braking systems. Before running equipment on roadways or a job site, make sure the roadway surface and slope are adequate for safe operation of the heavy equipment. Always enforce speed limits and load limits to ensure risks are mitigated.

REQUIRED TRAINING

Proper training is essential for employees who will operate heavy equipment. The training should start with formal classroom training to discuss the principles of operation, how the controls work, and what the safety considerations are. There should be instructor-led demonstrations of the equipment and practical exercises including behind-the-wheel practice in a controlled environment. Training should also cover how to mount and dismount the equipment as this is a common action that causes injury to heavy equipment operators. Training should also cover proper fueling techniques and how to use hand signals common in heavy equipment operation.

SPECIFIC PRECAUTIONS FOR FRONT-END LOADERS, EXCAVATORS, AND BACKHOES

Front-end loaders, excavators, and backhoes are used to move soil and rocks. The center of gravity of the unit changes according to the weight of the load carried, and the height of the load, creating a risk of tipping. When traveling with a load, the load should be kept as low as possible. Only use the machines for transporting soil and soil-like materials; for example, do not use a front-end loader to transport beams or other oddly-shaped materials. Drive forward when going uphill, and when turning corners with a load go slowly and pay attention to the possibility that the load may shift. When using a backhoe, always put the stabilizers down when digging to ensure the unit doesn't tip. With all types of machines, ensure that there is a stable digging platform before engaging in the excavation. Consult the machine's specifications to understand how much the unit can safely lift and under what conditions. Always wear a seat belt when operating heavy equipment.

HAZARDS AND CONTROLS ASSOCIATED WITH COMPRESSED GAS STORAGE AND USE
STORAGE

Compressed gas cylinders pose special hazards due to the high pressure in the cylinders in addition to any flammability hazard that may be posed by the gas itself. Cylinders that are struck or impacted may suddenly release pressure forcefully, causing the cylinder to move quickly and possibly strike someone in its path. Cylinders must be segregated according to incompatibilities (e.g., store oxygen away from acetylene). They must be stored securely in upright positions and constrained in a cage or rack that prevents them from falling over or from being inadvertently bumped. The valve cap must be on the cylinder to protect the valve when it is not in use.

CHANGING LIQUEFIED PETROLEUM GAS CYLINDERS ON FORKLIFTS

Changing liquefied petroleum gas (LPG) cylinders presents several hazards: flammability, skin damage from cold surfaces if contact with the LPG occurs, and potential eye hazards. There should never be any smoking or source of flame present when changing a cylinder. The cylinder to be changed should have the main valve closed before moving it. The employee should wear leather gloves and only use non-sparking tools to loosen bolts. Always take care not to dent or damage the cylinder. The cylinders (whether empty or full) should be stored securely in racks and not left sitting on the ground unsecured.

COMPRESSED GASES COMMONLY USED IN WELDING

There are several commonly used compressed gases used in welding processes. Compressed oxygen is used in many processes. The source of fuel for the welding process is commonly acetylene. Other commonly used gases in welding are hydrogen, helium, carbon dioxide, and argon. Several of these gases are flammable, oxygen is an oxidizer, and the welding process itself is a source of ignition; therefore, care must be taken to keep all ignitable items away from the welding process. Oxygen should be stored separately from the other gases and be separated by a firewall with at least a half-hour fire rating. Another peculiarity of welding gases applies to acetylene – acetylene cylinders should never be stored horizontally and if they have been, they must be stored upright for a minimum of an hour before the gas is used again.

INDUSTRIAL HYGIENE AND PERSONAL SAFETY RISKS

Compressed gas cylinders pose several physical hazards in addition to the exposure risks posed by the gases themselves. Care must be taken not to bump into or jostle the cylinders. They should always be stored upright and secured by a chain to prevent them tipping over. The caps should be screwed in place; they should not be stored with the access valve exposed. Exposure to welding gases in a confined space is an industrial hygiene hazard and a flammable hazard; for this reason, Teflon tape should always be used on the screw threads of the joints to prevent leaks. Any situation that causes the gas to be quickly released from the cylinder may make the cylinder into a rocket that can cause severe injury.

HAZARDS AND CONTROLS FOR AMMONIA

Anhydrous ammonia is caustic and corrosive and exists as a gas at standard temperatures and pressures; therefore, it must be stored and transported as a compressed gas. OSHA 29 CFR 1910.111 contains the regulations concerning anhydrous ammonia. Exposure to anhydrous ammonia causes severe burns and frostbite to eyes, skin and the respiratory system. Employees that work around anhydrous ammonia should not wear contact lenses, however, they should wear eye and face protection, and appropriate gloves. Ammonia storage systems must be constructed of steel instead of galvanized piping. Ammonia vapors can be flammable at concentrations of 15% - 28%; therefore, all sources of ignition must be eliminated if there is a possibility of concentrations in this range. All storage and transport systems must be equipped with pressure relief valves. Storage tanks should be painted with reflective white paint to keep the tank as cool as possible. During unloading, the delivery vehicle must have the brake set and the wheels chocked. Delivery hoses and lines must be properly bled before disconnecting to avoid exposure and release of ammonia.

HAZARDS AND CONTROLS ASSOCIATED WITH RADIATION

There are three types of radiation: alpha, beta, and gamma. Proper shielding is the best protection from the harmful effects of radiation.

Alpha radiation is made up of small, positively charged particles. Due to an alpha particle's size and characteristics, it cannot travel great distances and is easily stopped by clothing, gloves, or a piece of paper. Care must be taken not to breathe alpha particles into the lungs, as they will damage the lungs and potentially cause cancer.

Beta radiation has a higher energy level than alpha radiation and therefore a greater ability to penetrate surfaces. However, it can be easily blocked by a layer of aluminum foil or similar material.

Gamma radiation has the highest energy level and has the most ability to penetrate the human body. Lead is the most common shielding used for gamma radiation; several centimeters is usually sufficient to shield from gamma radiation. Water can also be used for shielding; nuclear reactors and power plants use water shielding. Several feet of water are needed to shield from gamma radiation.

NON-IONIZING RADIATION

OSHA defines **non-ionizing radiation** as a series of energy waves from electric and magnetic fields. As with other radiation sources, these types of radiation travel at the speed of light. There are several sources of non-ionizing radiation:

- Power lines, electrical equipment, and household electric wiring produce extremely low frequency (ELF) radiation.
- Radio frequency and microwave radiation may be absorbed through the skin and body. At high levels, this type of radiation can cause tissue damage due to the heating of the body. Radio transmitters and cell phones are examples.
- Infrared radiation is emitted from such sources as heat lamps and lasers that operate from this wavelength.
- Visible light radiation can damage eyes and skin if it is too intense. The visible light spectrum is what we normally see with our eyes.
- UV or ultraviolet radiation sources come from welding arcs and UV lasers.

IONIZING RADIATION

Ionizing radiation is radiation that can produce ions when it interacts with atoms and molecules. Types of ionizing radiation include x-rays, alpha particles, beta particles, gamma radiation, and neutrons. Ionizing radiation can come from natural sources, such as cosmic radiation and radioactive soils, and from artificial sources, such as television sets, diagnostic x-rays, and nuclear fuels. Exposure to ionizing radiation damages human cells, especially rapidly developing cells. It is especially dangerous for infants and children, who have the most rapidly developing cells. Exposure to high doses of ionizing radiation causes radiation sickness, characterized by weakness, sleepiness, stupor, tremors, convulsions, and eventually death. Low doses may cause more delayed effects, such as genetic effects, cancers, cataracts, and shortened life span.

PREVENTING DAMAGE

The damage caused by ionizing radiation depends on the type and dose of the radiation, the tissue and organs exposed, and the age of the person being exposed. The best way to control potential damage is to limit the amount of radiation people are exposed to by limiting the amount of source material. It is also important to limit the amount of time people are exposed to radiation. Other ways to reduce exposure to ionizing radiation include the following:

- Increasing the distance between people and sources of ionizing radiation.
- Using shielding such as air, hydrogen, and water to protect people from sources of radiation. The material used as a shield depends on the type of radiation.
- Using barriers such as walls and fences to keep people away from sources of radiation.
- Using liners and protective materials to keep contaminated waste from leaching into groundwater.

A key concept in radiation protection is to keep the radiation dose "as low as reasonably achievable" (ALARA). Regardless of whether the radiation is alpha, beta, or gamma particles, both time and distance can be used to reduce the amount of exposure. Work schedules should be arranged so that exposure time is limited. Reducing the time exposed to radiation reduces the absorbed dose in a directly proportional manner. Distance away from the radiation source can also be used as a means of reducing absorbed radiation. As one moves away from the radioactive source, the exposure decreases according to the inverse square of the distance, as illustrated by the following formula: intensity is proportional to $\frac{1}{x^2}$ where x is the distance from the radiation source.

SAFETY CONTROLS

Warnings need to mark any areas where ionizing radiation is located, as well as equipment that uses ionizing radiation. In addition to signs on these areas, flashing lights and audio signals can serve as additional warnings.

Evacuation is a tool used to remove people from an area where a significant amount of ionizing radiation has been released.

Security procedures need to be in place to keep sources of ionizing radiation from getting into the wrong hands. Procedures can include physical monitoring, controlled entry and exit, and manifest systems.

Dosimetry measures people's exposure to ionizing radiation. It is necessary because we cannot see or feel this radiation. People who work with or near ionizing radiation also need training about its hazards and how to protect themselves and others.

System design and analysis can help prevent dangerous exposure to ionizing radiation by anticipating and preventing possible sources of failure.

DECAY AND HALF-LIFE

Radioactive decay, or radioactivity, is a set of processes that allow unstable atomic nuclei, or nuclides, to emit subatomic particles, or radiation. Radioactive decay is a random process, and it is not possible to predict an individual atom's decay. However, on a larger scale, radioactive material behaves in a predictable manner. Radioactive decay occurs at an exponential rate. This means that the amount of radioactive material, N, present after time t is given by the following equation, where

N_0 is the amount of material present at time $t = 0$; e is the constant known as Euler's number, approximately 2.71828; and λ is the decay constant of the material:

$$N = N_0 e^{-\lambda t}$$

The time required for half the mass of a radioactive material to decay is known as its **half-life**. Half-life is the most commonly used measure of a material's rate of decay, and it can be as short as a fraction of a second or as long as millions of years. If the half-life of the material is known, then **lambda**, the decay constant, can be calculated as $\lambda = \frac{\ln(2)}{t_{1/2}}$, where $t_{1/2}$ is the half-life.

For example, suppose a sample of radium-224 starts at a mass of 10 grams. Its half-life is 3.63 days. The remaining mass of radium-224 after 8 days can be calculated by:

$$\lambda = \frac{\ln(2)}{3.63 \text{ days}} = 0.191 \text{ disintegrations per day}$$

$$N = 10e^{-0.191 \times 8} = 2.17 \text{g}$$

RADIOACTIVE WASTE

Radioactive waste is regulated by the Nuclear Regulatory Commission, a division of the US Department of Energy. Radioactive waste is classified differently than hazardous waste. Classification is according to the source of the material, with subdivisions based on the level of radioactivity.

- *High Level Waste* is derived from spent fuel rods or waste from reprocessing.
- *Transuranic Waste* contains uranium (atomic number 92) and elements of higher atomic number
- *Low Level Waste* is all other radioactive wastes. These are classified into Class A (average 0.1 curies/cubic ft), Class B (average 2 curies/cubic ft), Class C (average 7 curies/cubic ft) and GTCC (Greater Than Class C) (300 – 2500 curies/cu ft).

MOBILE PHONE USE IN THE WORKPLACE

BEST MANAGEMENT PRACTICES

Employers should consider the risks of mobile phone use particular to their workplace and implement a best management practice with regard to their use in the workplace. Use of cell phones for talking or texting should be prohibited when employees are operating any equipment (such as forklifts) or driving (whether they are in a company vehicle or a personal vehicle for company activities). Employers should not allow employees to walk while they are texting or e-mailing—they may trip, sprain an ankle when stepping off a curb, or run into an obstacle without seeing it. Employers should also consider the potential loss of productivity by use of mobile phones in the workplace and restrict the use.

HAZARDS

The hazards posed by use of mobile phones in the workplace are mostly centered on the distraction they cause. They are most hazardous when used by employees who are driving in the course of their employment; mobile phone use is already banned for commercial drivers, but employers must also be aware of the hazards mobile phone use poses to those who drive during work hours to appointments or customer sites. Even talking on the phone with a hands-free device is risky; of course, texting and e-mailing while driving must be strictly prohibited. Employers should also be aware that once the policy is written, it must be properly communicated to employees, and the employer must be able to produce evidence of such in case of lawsuits.

PROXIMITY ALARMS

Proximity sensors and alarms are non-contact devices used to warn employees when they are about to come into contact with a hazard. The most common application of a proximity alarm is in a forklift traffic environment where views and lines of sight may be obstructed. The forklift is equipped with a sensor and the employees working on foot in the area wear a sensor. When the sensor detects the presence of the forklift an alarm is sounded to provide warning. Proximity alarm systems can also be used to warn of hazards near an excavation, equipment with moving parts, or conveyors. Vehicles can be equipped with proximity sensors that detect solid objects; these can be used to prevent backing up into walls or other vehicles. Proximity sensors can also be used in machine guarding; for example, a light curtain can be used to detect the presence of an employee's hands entering an unsafe area. The sensor detects the break in the beam of light and shuts down the equipment before an injury occurs. Many automatic garage doors have this type of sensor.

TECHNICAL DRAWINGS AND DIAGRAMS

Technical drawings are used to show equipment layouts and to document products. In environmental health and safety, facility layout drawings are necessary to document emergency equipment locations and evacuation routes. They must also be submitted with environmental permit applications. For example, air permit applications will require drawings of process equipment and associated air pollution control equipment. Drawings are made 'to scale' which allows a reference for the spacing and relative size of equipment. "To scale" means that a certain length on the drawing corresponds to a certain length in reality. For example, the scale may be one inch on the drawing equals twenty feet in the physical world. The legend gives the meaning for the various symbols used. For example, the legend will define which lines represent pipes, paved roads, dirt roads, etc. Units of measurement, whether feet and inches or metric unites, will be indicated on the drawing.

PROCESS FLOW DIAGRAMS

Process flow diagrams are a way to visually communicate and document a manufacturing or other process flow. They are often submitted with environmental permit applications to illustrate the step-wise process for those that are unfamiliar with the process. They are used in process safety management to document each step in a process so that consideration can be given to potential hazards associated with each step. Process flow diagrams are also useful when there are many inputs and interrelated activities that need to be agreed upon by different functional units. Below are some symbols used in process flow diagrams:

- = Start or end of process
- = Decision Point
- = Data coming into or out of process
- = Document Step
- = Delay Step
- = Manual input step

BUILDING DESIGN AND CONSTRUCTION BASICS

Proper ventilation is important for employee comfort and health. For standard workspaces (those that contain no hazardous atmospheres), OSHA recommends that the air in the space be exchanged three to ten times per hour. This means the total air flowing out of and into the space is three to ten times the volume of the space each hour. Air can move in and out of the environment by passive diffusion through open doors and windows, or it can be mechanically forced by a heating and air conditioning system. In this case, the fresh air intake should not be located near a loading dock or other area that may potentially pull air with toxic fumes into the building. Ventilation requirements are increased for hazardous atmospheres or the presence of fine particulates. There may also be a need for additional local ventilation provided by vent hoods that pull air out of a particular space and vent it to the outside. Air removed from a hazardous environment cannot be re-circulated back into the environment if it contains things like lead or toxic organic vapors.

The International Building Code lists the requirements for occupancy ratings. Occupancy rating is based on the purpose and layout of the space. You calculate max occupancy using the total square footage of the space divided by the number of square feet required per occupant as found in the IBC manual. If the space has tables and chairs (like a restaurant) then the maximum occupancy is calculated by taking the total square footage of the space and dividing by 15 (which is the IBC requirement). If you had a restaurant with 1000 square feet filled with tables and chairs, the maximum occupancy would be 1000 divided by 15, yielding a max occupancy of 66 people (you always round down to the more conservative number of occupants). For a space where there is mostly standing (no tables and chairs) like a bar, then the IBC square footage per occupant is 7. You must also have enough exits. The minimum number of exits required is based on the occupancy load: 1-500 people = 2; 501-1,000 = 3; more than 1,000 = 4. There are other factors that would increase the required number of exits. Warehouses are rated at 500 square feet per person and manufacturing areas at 200 square feet per person. Therefore, a 10,000-square-foot manufacturing area would have a max occupancy of 50 people.

Health Hazards and Basic Industrial Hygiene

ERGONOMICS

Ergonomics is the study of the use of the human body in the work environment. It refers to how the body is configured, the motions it is required to take, and the forces applied to muscles and bones by the work. Ergonomics seeks to adapt the work demands to make them as easy as possible for the body to endure to prevent injury. Anyone who has participated in physical activities and been sore the next day understands the effects of overexertion. Overexertion at work over long periods of time can lead to injuries that can be costly to treat. Even in the absence of an injury situation, improved ergonomics can improve productivity and comfort in the workplace.

PROPER LIFTING TECHNIQUE

Use of proper lifting techniques can prevent back strains in the workplace. The goal of proper lifting is to put as little stress on the spine as possible. The spine is meant to be straight, and lifting with a bent, curved-over spine puts extreme stress on it, even if the weight lifted is relatively small. To properly lift, place the feet hip-distance apart, and face the object to be lifted. Squat to pick up the object, then pull the object close to the body at the waist to move it. Stand up, using the strong thigh muscles to accomplish the work of lifting. Do not twist the spine when lifting or moving the object. Reverse the process to put down the object. Peer assessments should be conducted regularly to reinforce proper lifting techniques as people tend to get lazy and revert to poor lifting techniques.

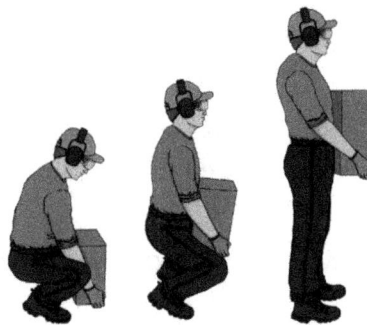

NEUTRAL SITTING POSTURE

A neutral sitting posture is important to prevent undue and fatiguing strain upon bones and muscles. Adjustments must be made to work table or desk height and chair height to achieve a neutral sitting posture. The chair should support the small of the back, and one should sit upright with the small of the back supported by the chair. Shoulders should be pulled back rather than hunched or tensed. The arms should hang from the shoulders in a relaxed manner, and the elbows should make a comfortable ninety-degree angle. The feet should be flat on the floor (no legs crossed), and the knees should also make a ninety-degree angle.

NEUTRAL STANDING POSTURE

A neutral standing posture can help prevent fatigue and muscle strain. The feet should be kept shoulder-width apart for optimal support. Shifting one's weight from one foot to the other is a sign of fatigue that indicates inattention to neutral standing posture. Hips should be in line with the

125

shoulders and the knees. The arms should hang comfortably at one's side, and the shoulders should not be hunched or tensed. The neck should stay straight (head not bent over), and the spine should stay straight, not twisted.

Repetitive Stress Injury

A repetitive stress injury is caused by using the same muscles, tendons, and bones repetitively several times over the course of a work day. Repetitive stress injuries occur because of strains on muscles, tendons, and ligaments. If caught early, and the stress is eliminated early, they are almost always reversible. However, repetitive stress injuries can also lead to employees having to have surgery and spend weeks away from work, followed by months of light duty. A common example of a repetitive stress injury is carpal tunnel syndrome, which is a disorder of the tendons and nerves in the wrists and hands experienced by some workers who must do repetitive work with their hands (such as data entry operators, typists, or hand assembly workers).

TECHNIQUES TO DECREASE LIKELIHOOD OF INJURY: Repetitive stress injuries are caused by using the same motion (and thus, the same muscle groups and bones) over and over again. Another contributing factor is the force applied to the motion. To reduce the likelihood, it is important to quantify the loads and the numbers of repetitions. Configure the work areas to ensure that items used most often are within close reach and that long reaches or limb extensions are only required infrequently. Break up loads into smaller weights. It is also important to evaluate whether employees' work stations are configured to ensure neutral postures are used most of the time. In addition, job rotation can also be important to changing the motions employees have to make over the course of the work day.

Minimizing or Eliminating Lifting Hazards

Minimizing or eliminating lifting hazards should be pursued as an effective injury prevention tool. Tools to do this include ensuring that all loads lifted with regularity are less than 25 pounds, and heavier loads that must be lifted must use a buddy system (two-person lift) or assistive device (forklift, drum lifter, or vacuum-powered lifter). Pallet jacks that can be height adjusted to the work level can minimize or eliminate the need to carry a package from floor height to work table height, which decreases the risks posed. Carts can be used to transport items that must be moved from one location to another rather than carrying them.

Computer Workstation Setup to Minimize Ergonomic Issues

A computer workstation in which the user will sit should be set up so that the head, hands, arms, wrists, and legs are in the most neutral position possible. Due to variation in height, each person should adjust his or her station to suit individual needs. The computer monitor should be at slightly below eye level so that the neck does not have to be bend to view it. The keyboard should be arranged so that one can type on it while keeping the wrists straight and the elbows at a comfortable 90-degree angle. The chair should be adjusted so that the feet rest flat on the floor and the knees remain at a 90-degree angle. The chair back should support the back and allow one to sit with the back resting on the support rather than slouched over. Items that are frequently used (such as the phone) should be within easy reach so that arm extension is not required to use them.

Carpal Tunnel Syndrome

Carpal tunnel syndrome is a painful condition marked by swelling and inflammation caused by compression of a major nerve that runs through the front of the wrist. It is characterized by a numbness, tingling, and burning sensation in the hands and may cause reduced grip strength. It is a controversial syndrome in that it has been attributed to repetitive motion of the hands (such as high-speed data entry); however, some researchers are beginning to determine other factors that

increase the likelihood of developing carpal tunnel syndrome, such as diabetes. Exercises that increase strength in the hands and wrists and promote blood flow can help prevent carpal tunnel syndrome, as can job rotation and proper ergonomics. Treatment generally involves rest, sometimes medications are prescribed, and surgery is also used to relieve the inflammation.

WORKPLACE LIGHTING

Workplace lighting is measured in "foot candles". Foot-candles can be measured with a simple light meter. OSHA has different foot-candle requirements for different types of worksite. The amount of illumination needed by workers is dependent upon the site itself. One foot-candle represents the amount of light upon a given surface at the rate of one lumen per square foot.

- General worksite areas require 5 foot-candles. 5 foot-candles is also the required illumination for indoor warehouses, corridors and hallways, etc.
- Mining operations have requirements which depend on location, ranging from 5-10 foot-candles.
- General worksite plant and shops require 10 foot-candles.
- Excavations, storage, maintenance, and loading areas require 3 foot-candles.
- Hospitals, first-aid stations, and offices require 30 foot-candles.

OCCUPATIONAL ILLNESSES
AIDS AND BLOODBORNE PATHOGENS

Procedures that can protect workers from AIDS and bloodborne pathogens in the workplace include the following:

- Treating all bodily fluids as if they are contaminated.
- Using self-sheathing needles, leakproof specimen containers, and puncture-proof containers for sharp objects.
- Providing handwashing stations with antiseptic hand cleaners and requiring workers to wash their hands after removing gloves that could be contaminated.
- Prohibiting employees from eating or drinking in areas where bloodborne pathogens could be present.
- Providing gloves, goggles, respirators, aprons, and other personal protective equipment.
- Regularly decontaminating and cleaning equipment and potentially contaminated areas.
- Labeling potential biohazards.

An AIDS and bloodborne pathogens policy should be developed before any employees test positive for a disease. Preparing in advance allows the company to spend time determining appropriate actions instead of having to react quickly. An AIDS and bloodborne pathogens policy needs to include at least three elements: employee rights, testing, and education. It should define the rights of employees who have been diagnosed with AIDS or a bloodborne pathogen, including reasonable accommodations that will be made. The policy will also include whether employees will be tested for AIDS and bloodborne pathogens. Finally, the policy should include procedures for educating workers on how AIDS and other bloodborne pathogens can be transmitted and prevented.

OTHER WORKPLACE ILLNESSES

Workplace illnesses often take the form of skin disorders. Other workplace illnesses may have a respiratory origin. Poisoning accounts for still other workplace illnesses. A partial list of workplace illnesses would include:

- Skin diseases: Eczema, dermatitis, blisters, rashes, or other inflammation may be caused by environmental factors. Exposure of uncovered body parts to concrete may, over time, result in a painful skin condition which limits or prevents working.
- Respiratory conditions: These are common environmental hazards in the workplace. Asbestosis, Silicosis ("Black Lung") TB, certain forms of asthma, COPD, and chronic obstructive bronchitis are just a few examples of respiratory diseases caused by tiny airborne particles.
- Poisoning: Harmful metals in the environment can be absorbed into the human body with disastrous results. Gases, metals, and solvents are often found in construction areas. Mercury, arsenic, cadmium and lead are poisonous components found commonly in old construction. Carbon monoxide poisoning can result from equipment motors and engines. Solvents like benzol or carbon tetrachloride are other examples of chemical poisons causing worker injury.

HAZARDS AND CONTROLS ASSOCIATED WITH NOISE

Noise is often measured in decibels (dB), but OSHA uses a slightly different scale, the A-weighted scale, dBA, that more closely matches the human ear's perception of sound. The most important thing to know about the decibel scale is that it is logarithmic, not linear. This means that an increase of ten decibels means that sound intensity (I) has been multiplied by 10. The sound intensity level (β) is calculated using the following equation, where β is sound intensity level (dBA), I is sound intensity (W), and I_0 is the reference sound intensity (10^{-12} W):

$$\beta = 10 \times \log\left(\frac{I}{I_0}\right)$$

Suppose there is a grinding machine that produces a sound intensity level of 60 dBA. The sound intensity can be calculated by:

$$I = I_0 \times 10^{\left(\frac{\beta}{10}\right)} = 10^{-12} \times 10^{\left(\frac{60}{10}\right)} = 10^{-6} \text{ W}$$

If a second identical machine is turned on, the sound intensity (I) will double, 2×10^{-6}. Plugging this new value into the sound intensity level (β) equation yields:

$$\beta = 10 \times \log\left(\frac{2 \times 10^{-6}}{10^{-12}}\right) = 63.01 \text{ dBA}$$

DETERMINING ADEQUATE LEVEL OF HEARING PROTECTION

The OSHA hearing conservation standard establishes a permissible exposure limit to noise at 90 decibels (dBA). Exposures above 90 dBA require employees to wear hearing protection in the form of muffs or earplugs. Hearing protection devices have a Noise Reduction Rating provided by the manufacturer. Theoretically, wearing the device reduces the noise exposure by that number of decibels. In practice, one applies a safety factor. This calculation requires the "A-weighted" sound-level readings from a noise meter (the A-level readings are expressed as "dBA" and represent the exposure as heard by the human ear, with very high and low frequencies screened out). The calculated employee exposure wearing the hearing protection is as follows:

$$\text{Estimated Exposure (dBA)} = \text{TWA (dBA)} - (\text{NRR} - 7)$$

If C-level noise readings are available, the Noise Reduction Rating can be subtracted directly from the dBC reading to determine estimated employee exposure.

CONTROL METHODS FOR EXPOSURE TO EXCESSIVE LEVELS OF NOISE

Engineering controls are the first consideration for control of excessive exposure to noise. Sound-dampening foam products can be used to line enclosures and dampen noise from machinery. Where noise can't be avoided, its effects can be reduced by grouping and enclosing noisy processes in a soundproof area so that people working in other areas are not bothered. Design features that can help reduce noise include the following:

- Controlling the direction of the source
- Reducing flow rates
- Reducing driving forces
- Controlling vibrating surfaces
- Using barriers and shields
- Building with sound-absorbing materials

In addition to controlling the noise source itself, you can also protect the workers by requiring **protection** such as earplugs or earmuffs.

RESPIRATOR HAZARDS AND CONTROLS

An inhalation hazard is a toxic material that presents a hazard to human health when breathed into the lungs. These substances are injurious to mucous membranes that line the nasal passages and lungs, or otherwise react quickly to enter the bloodstream and cause an adverse reaction. Inhalation hazards may be in the form of gases or aerosolized substances that can be breathed in. Examples of inhalation hazards include organic vapors such as solvents. The US DOT definition of inhalation toxicity is more specific. It is defined as a substance that is a dust or mist with an LC_{50} for acute toxicity upon inhalation of less than or equal to 10 mg/L or a material with a saturated vapor concentration in air at 20°C (68°F) of more than one-fifth of the LC_{50} for acute toxicity on inhalation of vapors and with an LC_{50} for acute toxicity on inhalation of vapors of less than or equal to 5000 ml/m³.

RESPIRATOR CARTRIDGES

Respirator cartridges are specific to particular respiratory hazards. The manufacturers of respirator cartridges publish charts that can be consulted to ensure that the right cartridge is chosen for the hazard. Respirator cartridges are available for gases and vapors (organic gases, ammonia, acid gases, for mercury vapor) and for particulates. Cartridges are also available for a combination of the gases and vapors and the particulates. The particulate filter efficiencies range from 95 percent to 99 percent to 99.97 percent efficient at removing particles down to a certain micron size. It is important to choose the correct filter for the hazard that is present; if a respirator cartridge is not available for the specific hazard, then an SCBA will have to be considered (assuming there is no engineering control available.) It is also important to specify a respirator cartridge change schedule; this can be determined empirically or by using an e-Tool available at the OSHA website.

RESPIRATOR PRE-USE REQUIREMENTS

According to the OSHA Respiratory Protection Standard, **e**mployees who are required to wear respirators at work (either half-mask, full face, or self-contained breathing apparatus) must be given a spirometry (lung function) test and be evaluated by an occupational health physician to determine their fitness to wear a respirator. Then, training on the airborne hazard must be given, along with information about the following:

- how a respirator works
- the limitations of the respirator
- how to determine whether the positive and negative qualitative fit test is passed
- how to tell when the cartridges need to be replaced
- how to clean and care for the respirator

COMMON OCCUPATIONAL INJURIES

OSHA defines a work-related injury as one that occurs in the work environment and was caused by an activity in the workplace which was performed as a condition of employment. An injury is *not* work-related when:

- The injured person is not an employee of the company.
- The symptoms of injury appear in the workplace while the cause of the injury occurred outside the workplace.
- The person is injured in voluntary recreational activity.
- The injury occurs outside working hours through voluntary activity not directed by the employer or related to employment.
- The injury is caused by motor vehicle accident during a commute to or from work.
- Common cold and flu are not considered work-related. (Contagious diseases like TB may be considered work-related if the employee contracted the disease while working at a jobsite as a condition of employment.)
- Mental illness is not considered work related unless that is determined and adequately documented by a licensed mental health care practitioner.

Categorizing a work-related incident as an injury or an illness can be confusing since both categories can occur in the workplace. Typically, an injury stems from a workplace event such as a slip, trip, or a fall or any physical activity which plays a major part in the occurrence of injury.

- Fractures, cuts, abrasions, contusions, and accidental amputations are injuries caused by falling, tripping, bumping or other general physical movements.
- Electrocution, thermal, and chemical burns have an immediate and visible injurious effect upon the body and are prime examples of work injury.
- Injuries like sprains, muscle tears, joint and connective tissue damage often occur due to lifting, stretching, or applying bodily force to heavy objects. These also fall into the category of workplace injury.
- An insect or animal bite is also classified as an injury though this is not caused by a physical action like lifting or falling.

ACUTE AND CHRONIC HEALTH HAZARDS

An acute health hazard is one that is immediate and occurs a short time after the exposure or trigger event. An example of an acute health effect is losing consciousness after overexposure to solvent fumes such as ether or experiencing shortness of breath after exposure to acid gas fumes. A chronic health hazard is one that occurs after exposure repeatedly over long time periods. An example of a chronic health hazard is overexposure to noise repeatedly during the work day over years that leads to hearing loss or exposures to low levels of benzene leading to cancer many years or decades later. The time between exposure and the appearance of an effect is known as the latency period and can be as long as 40 years.

HAZARDS AND CONTROLS REGARDING BIOLOGICAL SAFETY AND CONTAINMENT
BIOLOGICAL SAFETY LEVELS
There are four Biological Safety levels (BSL), in increasing order of risk. For all levels, standard laboratory precautions apply, such as no eating or drinking in the laboratory, wearing protective lab coats, wearing eye protection, and always washing hands after working in the lab. The four levels are:

Level 1 – This is the lowest BSL level. At this level, lab techs are dealing with biological agents that pose minimal hazard and are biological agents that do not normally cause human illness. Normal PPE and restrictions apply. An example of a Level 1 agent is strains of e. coli that are not pathogenic.

Level 2 – All of level 1 safety is in effect, plus: lab personnel have greater training; they are working with infectious agents. When these are aerosol or splashes are possible, then biological safety cabinets are used. Extreme precautions are used with contaminated sharp objects. An example of a Level 2 agent is HIV and staphylococcus aureus.

Level 3 – BSL-1 and BSL-2 are followed along with these protocols: Medical surveillance for lab personnel and immunization where available; all procedures are done within biological safety cabinets; solid front protective clothing is necessary. These are necessary because at this level the lab is working with microbes that can cause lethal disease through inhalation. These laboratories must be specially designed to contain agents and have special ducted ventilation. Examples of agents that are classified as Level 3 include yellow fever, west Nile virus, and tuberculosis bacteria.

Level 4 – is the highest level of biosafety. This classification is for dangerous agents that are usually fatal and have no available vaccine such as the Ebola and Marburg viruses. All work in a Level 4 facility must be conducted inside a level III biological containment cabinet or a level II Biological containment unit while wearing a positive pressure suit. When exiting all personnel must pass through a chemical decontamination shower and an airlock.

BIOSAFETY STORAGE CABINETS
Biosafety storage cabinets are designed and certified according to NSF standards. There are three levels of biosafety cabinet. Both I and II are suitable for low and moderate risk biological agents that can be handled in biosafety laboratories designated as Level 1, Level 2 and Level 3. A Level I biosafety cabinet does not isolate the product stored in it from the room ventilation, so may contaminate the product with room air (and vice versa). A Level II biosafety cabinet does filter the air supply going into the cabinet from the room air with a HEPA filter, and so protects the product stored, the personnel in the room or area, and the environment from contamination. A Level III biosafety cabinet is the highest level of protection, and applies to a Level 4 biosafety laboratory. These are gas-tight, completely sealed cabinets with a viewing window. There is no chance of contamination or communication of air or substances between what's stored in the cabinet and the laboratory environment. Both the supply air and the exhaust air are filtered, providing the maximum level of containment.

SHARPS MANAGEMENT

Sharps refer to needles that have been used to deliver intravenous medicine and scalpels that are potentially contaminated with human blood. If one is punctured or cut with a used needle or scalpel, diseases such as hepatitis or HIV can be transmitted. Best practices require an evaluation to determine if a needleless product is available to accomplish the task. Prompt disposal of all sharps is necessary; do not leave them unattended in the work area. Needles should not be broken or sheared off. Needles should not be re-capped by holding the cap in one hand and the needle in the other, as this poses a needle-stick hazard. Containers used for sharps disposal must be puncture-resistant and leak proof. The sharps container must not be overfilled and kept closed except when adding to the container.

LOCAL EXHAUST VENTILATION

For those locations where high volumes of toxic or hazardous materials are the result of some manufacturing or processing procedure, local exhaust ventilation is needed. While general ventilation controls the airflow throughout a structure, local exhaust only deals only with a specific location in order to capture and vent the unwanted air. A well-designed facility will isolate the area where the toxic or hazardous contaminants are generated and use local exhaust to completely ventilate the area and provide for a healthy work environment for employees. The local exhaust system will handle both large and small quantities of generated hazards through an exhaust hood designed for the airflow capacity needed. The major drawback to local exhaust ventilation system is the cost and specificity of the system to the location and purpose.

STRESS-RELATED CONDITIONS AND RESPONSES

WORKPLACE VIOLENCE

Managers can incorporate several strategies into the workplace to prevent or reduce **workplace violence** and provide a secure workplace.

- The workplace should be well-lit, with no areas that are secluded or isolated.
- Workflows and traffic patterns should be easily observed so employees are never left in a vulnerable position. Employees should have freedom and control within their own area of the workplace but limited access to other areas.
- Surveillance cameras can allow for further monitoring of the workplace.
- Employers can also control access to the workplace. Fencing and locks can restrict trespassers from entering the work area. Security procedures that require visitors to check in reduce the risk of violence from outsiders.

WORKPLACE STRESS

Stress is defined as the body's response to perceived threats. Stress can result in emotional problems such as anxiety and aggression, behavioral problems such as clumsiness and trembling, or cognitive problems such as problems concentrating or making decisions. Workplace stress is a serious problem, costing over $150 billion dollars a year. In fact, more than 15 percent of workplace disease claims are stress-related. In addition to contributing to accidents and injuries, stress is also linked to lower productivity, excess absenteeism and turnover, and poor morale. Workplace stress generally stems from a poor fit between the employee and the job. Specific issues can be poor physical working conditions, too much work or tasks that are too complex, lack of feedback or control over job responsibilities, unpredictable work schedules, and tense work relationships. In addition, personal and family problems can also contribute to workplace stress.

LOSS OF CONSCIOUSNESS

An employee that loses consciousness should be given immediate first aid. If a spinal injury is suspected, care must be taken not to move the head and neck. In the case of an unresponsive adult that is not breathing, call 911 to summon emergency assistance immediately. Give first aid by opening the airway to facilitate breathing. Open the air way and give two rescue breaths; commence administering cardiopulmonary resuscitation (CPR). Only trained individuals should administer CPR. If the unresponsive adult is breathing on his own, and if no spinal cord injury is suspected, place the individual in the 'recovery' position (on his side). Emergency medical services (911) should be called for anyone that does not regain consciousness within a minute. Tight clothing and a belt can be loosened to facilitate breathing.

INDUSTRIAL HYGIENE SAMPLE AND INDICATOR MEDIA

There are three basic types of sampling methods used to determine concentration levels of gases and vapors: a spot-check or snapshot sample, a long-term sample, and a passive sample. A spot-check is a quick sample of the air in a specific location which is good for determining exposure risk at the moment of the sample. A more thorough evaluation of the air environment for long-term exposure is the long-term sample where a device samples the air over a period of time of eight hours or more to determine the contamination level for an average work day or the length of the sample. The passive sample method is where a worker wears a sample device that simply warns when contamination levels are too high. Although the passive sample seems like the simplest method for keeping workers out of harm's way, these devices provide no measurement capability for preventive measures.

Sampling for particulates is a difficult task that requires an accurate determination of the type of sampling device to use. One must consider the type of measurement desired, the total concentration of a substance, or the concentration that poses an inhalation hazard. This distinction is needed because not all devices measure the smaller size particulates that pose inhalation hazards. The hygienist must also consider the particulate being measured and its characteristics, like water solubility or a tendency to clump, which will determine the type of sampling method used for accurate readings. If a substance will dissolve in a liquid, sampling methods that employ liquids should not be used. If the particulates tend to compact and the measurement requires a true reading of individual particles and their definition or shape, a deep filter should not be used.

Centrifugal Separators are effective for collecting measurements of larger particles because they use a centrifuge to separate particles by size. Electrostatic Precipitators are best used by large power plants to control aerosols and are also efficient for measuring particulate matter but cause an electric field with a corona discharge, which produces ozone. Elutriators collect particles as they naturally settle and usually collect a larger sample of the heavier particles. Filtration is most common which uses a filter along with an air-flow indicator and a pump. Impactors use an impact plate to capture particulates as they travel with the air flow measuring the captured particulates. Impingers, similar to impactors, add a liquid medium to the plate to trap matter. Piezoelectric Sensors use a vacuum to pull particles into a chamber where two sensors measure the weight of the particles and the air conditions present to determine the concentration of the particulate matter.

COLORIMETRIC INDICATOR TUBES

Colorimetric indicator tubes are a popular method for monitoring for airborne contaminants since the tubes provide a quick response and are easy to use. The tubes work by drawing a certain amount of air through the tube, passing through a layer of cotton and a conditioning filter, then interacting with an indicator ruler which changes color according to the concentration, and then back out through another cotton plug. The color changing indicator line is read against a direct reading scale which displays the concentration usually in parts per million. The colorimetric indicator tubes provide an excellent warning signal for certain hazardous contaminants and can be used for monitoring for several different chemicals, but the calibration of the tubes is a concern as only the manufacturer can do so, making inaccurate readings a higher risk factor. Once used, these tubes must be disposed of as hazardous waste.

PH STRIPS

pH is a scale from 1 – 14 that is a measure of acidity (free hydrogen ions in solution) or alkalinity (free hydroxyl ions in solution). pH strips are plastic or paper strips coated with a substance that changes color based on the amount of hydrogen or hydroxyl ions in a solution. Pure water is considered neutral with a pH of 7. pH strips can be used for quick determination of alkalinity or acidity of a liquid. If the pH is below 2 or above 12 then it is classified as a corrosive hazardous substance. pH strips are used on storm water runoff for monitoring purposes. pH analysis has a fifteen-minute holding time, which is not long enough to get a sample to the laboratory, making the test strip a useful alternative. pH determinations for regulatory compliance should ultimately be confirmed by use of a calibrated pH meter. pH strips must be protected from humidity and other gases to maintain accuracy.

SAMPLING EQUIPMENT

Below are several hand-held and portable instruments that are used in industrial hygiene applications:

Noise meters and dosimeters- are used to conduct sound level exposure surveys, and are worn for an entire shift to determine whether the OSHA Permissible Exposure Limit of 85 decibels was exceeded. Results and reports can be downloaded to a computer for storage and documentation.

Gas meters –are used for real-time analysis of various gas levels, such as, oxygen, carbon monoxide, and hydrogen sulfide. These are mandatory for permit-required confined space entry.

Gas detection tubes – are glass tubes containing a chemical-specific reactive substance used to measure concentrations of chemicals in the atmosphere. They are available for a variety of chemicals used in industry and provide an accurate assessment of exposure. Some are designed to be used with a hand-held pump and others are worn by the employee and sample the air by passive diffusion.

Photoionization detectors – are portable hand-held instruments that measure the concentration of volatile organic compounds in the air. They are not chemical-specific but measure all VOCs in the surrounding air. Photoionization detectors provide a way to assess exposure levels and establish level of respiratory protection needed in a given environment.

LIGHT METERS

Light is measured in units of lux, which is one lumen per square meter. A lumen is the intensity of one candle in a cone-shaped area. Light levels can be measured with hand-held instruments. Appropriate light levels are important for various tasks in order to reduce eye strain and avoid injury. To get a sense of the scale of lux values, a bright summer day is about 100,000 lux, an overcast summer day is about 1,000 lux, and twilight is about 10 lux. In occupational settings, a normal office environment should be at 250 – 500 lux. A supermarket or mechanical workshop should be approximately 750 lux. Detailed drawing work requires 1,500 – 2,000 lux for comfort. Consideration should also be given to the type of light used, as different types have different qualities. Light bulbs come in incandescent, fluorescent, and LED.

SOUND LEVEL METERS

There are two basic types of noise metering instruments available for onsite noise measurement to ensure compliance with OSHA noise regulations:

- General area noise meters are designed to measure the noise level in the areas where they have been placed. These instruments may be moved to other areas but have the disadvantage of providing only generalized data. Workers are often moving through a construction site where the noise levels vary according to the types of activity and machinery being used. A generalized metering scheme provides little data about the individual exposure record.
- Personal Noise Meter devices are designed to be worn by working personnel. Personal noise meters obtain individual readings. This type of noise metering has a practical advantage since it is common for workers to move through various work areas with different levels of noise production.

CONSTANT-FLOW SAMPLING PUMPS

Direct reading instruments take snapshots of the air quality and provide almost instant readings of the concentration levels of specified contaminants in the air. These readings are reliable enough for detection and early warning of possible hazardous exposure levels of the contaminants, but for complete accuracy and regulatory compliance verification, the constant flow sample pump is the measurement device used by OSHA. The constant flow air pump draws a measured amount of air through a filter medium for a given period of time to measure exposure levels for up to eight hours in a single day. The contaminants captured by the filter medium are analyzed by a laboratory to measure the concentration and determine the time-weighted exposure levels. This most accurate measurement of the contaminant level is used to determine whether or not a facility is in compliance with OSHA permissible exposure level limits regulated by OSHA.

RADIATION COUNTERS

There are several different methods and devices for detecting and determining exposure levels of ionizing radiation. Common devices used to determine exposure to individuals are dosimeters or film badges which are worn by the person. When exposed to ionizing radiation elements within the film react and when developed result in a permanent radiation exposure record. Dosimeters similarly react to the ionizing radiation and register a measurement of the exposure and in the case of a pocket dosimeter, which uses an ionization chamber, can be read immediately. Ionization chambers measure radiation exposure by the conductivity created by interaction of radiation with the enclosed gas. These chambers are used by themselves, in dosimeters, and are modified for use in Geiger-Mueller Counters. Scintillation instruments, which use phosphors or crystals to produce light in reaction to radiation, have been found to be extremely sensitive and useful when detecting low levels of exposure.

PASSIVE VS. ACTIVE SAMPLING EQUIPMENT

Passive air sampling equipment reads the molecular diffusion of the air without any powered assistance. The advantages of passive sampling are its low cost and ease of use. Active sampling equipment uses a pump to move air through the device. Cassettes or other means are used to trap particulates, aerosols, and other gases for testing. Using active sampling devices involves more training, but yields better and more precise results. It is critical to know what is being tested for and to develop a plan in advance to do this accurately. An example of using passive air sampling would be analyzing for ammonia vapors. The passive air sampling device contains tubes with chemicals that change color according to the amount of ammonia gas present. An example of active sampling would be testing for the quantity of lead particles suspended in the atmosphere in an area. The

135

sampling pump measures the total volume of air pulled through the sampling cassette. The particulates that are captured on the sampling cassette are analyzed and the total micrograms of lead divided by the volume of air in cubic meters determines exposure levels.

MEDICAL SURVEILLANCE

It is important to ensure that hazard control measures have been implemented and work effectively. One method of doing so is performing medical analysis on employees working with or around the hazards in question. For example, a hearing test can help determine if an employee stationed near a loud machine is exposed to too much noise. If the test shows that such an employee has slightly worse hearing than he did last month, it is likely that the noise abatement measures in place are insufficient. Using this information, the safety officer can recommend better ear protection for employees stationed near that machine, or a barrier between the work area and machinery. Medical surveillance allows preventative action to be taken before more serious issues develop.

Emergency Preparedness, Fire Prevention, and Security

TECHNIQUES FOR CONDUCTING AND EVALUATING EMERGENCY DRILLS AND EXERCISES

Emergency preparedness drills should be conducted for all employees at least once a year. Employees should be trained on emergency signals, evacuation procedures, location of assembly points, and appointing someone who is responsible for making sure all employees and visitors are accounted for. The supervisors and managers must receive a report showing that all workers and visitors have been accounted for and properly evacuated from the area. Employees also need to be trained on the all clear signal to let them know it is safe to return to work after an emergency. Post drill evaluations are critical to determine if the training has been effective and where additional training may be necessary. Spill response drills are another critical area of training. This drill ensures that personnel know their responsibilities during a hazardous spill. Those responsible should be trained on the location and proper use of spill remediation tools and supplies. Drills supplement education because it provides hands-on training to help personnel respond effectively to emergencies.

FIRE DRILLS

Conducting regular fire drills is an essential part of emergency planning. Fire drills can be announced or unannounced, but unannounced drills will provide a better gauge of how prepared and informed the staff actually is to carry out their duties during an emergency. When planning for a drill, contact the fire alarm company to alert them of the day and time of the drill so that emergency personnel are not notified. Activate the building fire alarm system, and have the supervisors or other designated emergency team members ensure that their areas are evacuated. The designated members of the team should sweep the areas to ensure that all personnel have evacuated. Roll call should be taken in the evacuation areas to ensure that all team members are accounted for. Once the drill is finished, the emergency response team should meet to debrief and consider what went well and where improvements in process or communication should occur. Finally, it is important to document the occurrence of the drill, the debriefing meeting, and actions for the record.

EMERGENCY EQUIPMENT USE AND INSPECTION

Regular inspection of emergency equipment is critical. Inspecting and maintaining emergency equipment ensure it is available and functional when needed. Below are several types of emergency equipment with inspection frequencies:

- **Fire extinguishers** – should be checked monthly to ensure they are fully charged, and serviced annually by the supplier.
- **Fire sprinkler systems** – Different aspects of the complete system should be tested quarterly, annually, and at five-year intervals.
- **Spill kits** – should be checked monthly to ensure they are staged in the proper areas and fully stocked.
- **PPE** – various according to type. But most should be checked monthly. Emergency PPE may include protective suits, gloves, respirators, and face shields.
- **Emergency lighting** – should be checked once a month to ensure it is functioning properly.
- **First aid kit** – should be checked once a month for low hazard industries, weekly for high hazard industries. They should be inspected to be sure they are fully stocked and up to date.

137

- *Fire and evacuation alarms* – should be tested annually, and annual drills should be conducted to ensure employees know where the assembly areas are located and what the emergency evacuation procedures are.

ORGANIZATIONAL AND COMMUNITY RESPONSE PLANS
FIRE SERVICE AND MUTUAL AID AGREEMENTS

In the United States, publicly funded fire departments are responsible for the majority of fire-related duties. Responsibilities of public fire departments include fire prevention and suppression as well as compelling compliance with ordinances and laws related to fire services. These departments often offer informative seminars and training for members of the community. This can range from fire prevention tips to CPR certification. All members of the community depend on service from public departments, including residential, commercial, and large-scale industrial. It is also common for companies, especially with large operations, to designate employees who lead in the area of fire safety. This role can include training other employees, performing routine inspections for fire hazards, and conducting fire drills. Mutual aid agreements are reached between fire service providers, stipulating that they will help one another in emergencies. This can benefit both groups by reducing the costs associated with labor and equipment.

BUSINESS CONTINUITY PLANS

A business continuity plan is a written document that plans for continued business operation and provision of services during interruptions due to natural disasters, fires, or pandemic disease outbreaks. A robust business continuity plan has input from operations, upper management, finance, human resources, safety, information technology, and logistics. First consideration should be given to the potential types of disasters, such as fire, flood, tornado, hurricane, earthquake, terror attack, or widespread power or other utility disruption. Critical supplier disruption should also be considered; for example, what alternative suppliers are available? Plans should be made for employee notification, customer notification, restoration of computer systems, restoration of the supply chain, and restoration of transport networks. The documents and telephone contact information should be kept in several locations on and off site and electronically accessible to the management team.

COMMUNITY RESPONSE PLANS

The following is a list of the key components of a robust Community Response Plan, including web resources:

1. Work with individuals in the community to help them identify disaster risks and develop a home/work plan. The plan should include an assessment of the following:
   a. Fire Safety
   b. Hazardous Materials
   c. Natural disasters
   d. Local industrial accidents
   e. Terrorist/chemical release disasters
2. Communicative Disease Outbreaks First response teams, protocols, and locations for medical assistance during a disaster, such as:
   a. Personal protection and medical hygiene for response teams
   b. Triage protocols
   c. Transport services
   d. Treatment locations
3. Train response teams to recognize possible psychological impact from trauma

4. Develop and train search and rescue teams
5. Websites:
   a. https://www.citizencorps.gov
   b. http://www.fema.gov/

COMMUNITY RIGHT-TO-KNOW

"Community Right to Know" is part of the Emergency Planning and Community Right to Know Act (EPCRA) of 1986. This federal law contains regulations that require companies that use or store toxic chemicals to make that information known to their community. There are four sections found in 40 CFR Part 350 – 372, as follows:

- **Emergency Planning** – requires companies that use, store, or generate hazardous chemicals to create emergency response plans and share those plans with local authorities.
- **Emergency Release Notification** – if release of a hazardous chemical to air, land, or water occurs in excess of the reportable quantity (RQ), notice must be made to the local authorities. The notice must also include measures that will be taken to contain and remediate spill/release.
- **Hazardous chemical storage reporting** – This is also known as hazardous materials business planning. Businesses are required to report to their local authority (usually the fire department, but it can be other agencies) the quantity and location of hazardous materials stored on-site, and to provide safety data sheets to local authorities for reference. This information can be used by first responders in the event of an emergency.
- **Toxic Chemical Release Inventory (TRI)** – This section requires companies in covered SIC codes to report releases to air (both stack and fugitive, planned and unplanned), water (wastewater and storm water), and land (wastes, including recycling) of hazardous chemicals that are manufactured or used in a process.

DEVELOPING COMPREHENSIVE EMERGENCY, CRISIS, AND DISASTER PLANS

Developing a comprehensive disaster plan can be accomplished by approaching the task in a planned fashion. First, a cross-functional disaster planning team should be assembled from various functions. The different viewpoints and areas of expertise will serve to strengthen the resulting plan. The next step is for the team to determine the range of disasters that should be planned for; in considering this list, it is important to begin the discussion locally and extend it out regionally and nationally. In addition, the team must consider all types of disasters, including natural, man-made, cybersecurity, and pandemic outbreaks. The team should create an overall disaster response outline, and then this overall scenario should be tailored for each considered disaster to take into account unique requirements. In each case, the team should consider how lines of communication will work, the government agencies that will need to be involved, and any specialized equipment that should be on hand to respond to the crisis. Finally, the team should consider who should be notified of the plan.

ANTICIPATING AND PLANNING FOR EMERGENCIES

The types of emergencies to plan for in an emergency response plan differ somewhat depending on geography, but all emergency response plans should plan for facility response in the case of a fire. The plan should list emergency response personnel phone numbers, and should document the steps the facility employees take in an emergency, and where they should assemble until given the all-clear signal. Additional emergencies to plan for include oil spills and chemical releases, earthquakes, and severe weather such as hurricanes or tornadoes. The plan should document the emergency equipment available in the facility such as fire-suppression systems and specialized personal protective equipment. Facilities should record the results of any emergency drills conducted so that the response actions can be evaluated to identify opportunities for improvement. Copies of the emergency response plan should be provided to local agencies responsible for emergency response, and in the case of facilities that have highly toxic or complex processes, the emergency response agency should visit to familiarize itself with the facility.

EARTHQUAKES

Earthquakes are most common in California, and there are also significant earthquake faults in the Pacific Northwest. Although strong earthquakes may only occur every 20 to 50 years, preparedness is essential. Again, prepare an emergency kit as for other disaster preparedness scenarios. If an earthquake hits, there is generally no warning. Stay inside, and do not stand in doorways. Get down on hands and knees to minimize the danger of falling over, and protect the head and neck from falling debris. Stay away from windows and objects that can fall. If outdoors, duck and cover, or get inside a building if possible.

TORNADOES

Tornadoes are common in the Midwest and into the Southeast of the United States. They can occur with little to no warning and cause localized, severe damage. Ensure you have an emergency kit if you are in one of these areas. Listen to the radio for tornado warnings and updates. Be aware of approaching storms and the factors that indicate conditions are favorable for the development of tornadoes: a dark sky, large hail, low-lying and rotating cloud formations, and a loud roar. Get into a designated safe room or basement to protect yourself. If a basement is not available, go to a small interior room, and stay away from windows. If outside, get into a vehicle for shelter; do not park under an overpass, and never try to outrun a tornado in your vehicle.

HURRICANES AND TROPICAL STORMS

Hurricanes and tropical storms are common in the Southeast of the country, especially along the Gulf Coast. Planning for these types of emergencies is similar to that for other types with regard to ensuring one has an emergency kit containing flashlights, batteries, nonperishable food, cash, necessary medication, and a radio for communication. However, there is usually sufficient warning that a hurricane may approach and authorities may call for evacuations. Although the exact path and strength of a hurricane or tropical storm cannot always be predicted, always evacuate if ordered to do so. Know the designated hurricane evacuation routes. Even if you don't need to evacuate, you must prepare for several days without power after a storm as infrastructure can be damaged and can take some time to repair.

TYPES OF FIRE SUPPRESSION SYSTEMS

There are several types of fire suppression systems available. The advantages and disadvantages of the four main types are as follows:

Dry Pipe Systems – have no water in the pipes. Water flows into the system when the response is triggered. This type of system is slower to respond in an emergency, but is used when the possibility of leaking or frozen pipes is a concern. There will be residual moisture in the system after testing that must be removed to decrease corrosion in the pipes.

Wet Pipe Systems – These are the most common type of system. Water stays in the pipes at all times. A heat-sensing mechanism triggers the valves and sprinkler heads to activate.

Deluge – In this system, the sprinkler heads are all open at all times but the pipes are dry. The system is connected to fire alarms triggered by smoke or heat sensors. It can also be manually engaged. It is good for suppressing fires in large areas or where spills of flammable materials are likely.

Pre-action – This type of system is used in cases where accidental activation is undesirable or detrimental (like libraries or computer centers). This system permits confirmation of an actual fire in these sensitive areas prior to activation.

BASIC FIRST AID
OSHA REQUIREMENTS

OSHA regulations require that all workplaces make provisions for providing employees with first aid response (29 CFR 1910.151). This means that first aid supplies must be on hand to address minor cuts and related first aid situations. Employers should also have on staff personnel who have basic first aid and CPR training. OSHA does not require any certain individual to perform first aid against their will, and employers cannot force a person to administer or to accept first aid. First aid is classified as minor medical care that can be performed with over-the-counter medicines (available without a prescription) and that do not require a physician to perform. First aid treatment also does not result in lost work time or restricted job duties.

CUTS

Basic first aid for cuts should aim to stop bleeding, disinfect the cut, and protect the cut from exposure to the elements. If the cut is bleeding, use a clean, sterile gauze pad to cover the cut, and firmly apply pressure until bleeding stops. Gently clean around the cut with antiseptic soap (the cut may begin bleeding again; if so, use a new gauze piece to apply pressure again). Apply antibiotic ointment to the cut, and bandage with a sterile bandage to protect the cut. Cuts do heal faster if protected from exposure to air and to friction. Be aware of the risk of infection; clean and bandage the cut daily. If the area becomes tender, red, and swollen, there may be an infection beginning that will require medical attention.

BURNS

Basic first aid for burns is similar to that for cuts. Basic first aid should only be applied to minor burns; burns that are greater than second degree require medical attention, and so do second-degree burns if they are large. First aid for minor burns involves keeping the burned area protected with a loosely applied, clean, sterile dressing such as a gauze pad. Do not apply ointments or creams to the burn. Be vigilant for signs of infection at the burn site, which is indicated by redness and swelling. There are also spray-on burn treatments that can be applied to assist in soothing the area and help the area to heal.

STRAINS

Strains occur when muscles are overstretched or overworked. As a result, muscles become inflamed and painful to move. Many times, strains can get better using first aid treatment and do not require a trip to the doctor. First aid for strains is best remembered by the RICE acronym:

- Rest the affected area.
- Ice the affected area for 20 minutes each hour, making sure to protect the skin from direct contact with the ice pack.
- Compress the affected muscle using an Ace bandage, making sure that it is not wound so tightly that it affects blood flow.
- Elevate the affected area above the heart if possible, to decrease swelling.

In addition, over-the-counter non-steroidal anti-inflammatory medication may be taken for the pain and swelling.

EMERGENCY FIRST AID EQUIPMENT AND PROCEDURES

EYEWASHES AND SAFETY SHOWERS

OSHA requirements for emergency eyewashes and showers are found in 29 CFR 1910.151. Requirements for eyewashes and showers are similar. They are required in areas where an employee might be exposed to corrosive or hazardous chemicals, such as strong acids or bases. Eyewashes and showers are required in work areas with anhydrous ammonia and forklift battery charging stations. The path to the eyewash or shower must be unobstructed, and require no more than 10 seconds of travel time from the hazard. Both eyewashes and showers must deliver tepid water. The flow must be able to be sustained for a minimum of fifteen minutes, and the valve that delivers the water must stay open on its own and not shut off unless someone physically shuts it off.

FIRE EXTINGUISHERS

OSHA regulations require a written fire prevention plan that is communicated to all employees (29 CFR 1910.39). Employers with fewer than ten employees may verbally tell their employees the plan. The plan must list the fire hazards present in the workplace, and procedures to control accumulation of flammable and combustible materials. There must be written procedures for maintenance of heat-producing equipment to prevent accidental build-up of heat and ignition of combustible materials. Part of the fire prevention plan must describe where fire extinguishers are located, and what type of fire extinguisher is appropriate for the fire hazard. Fire extinguishers should be located near areas with fire hazards. Employees must receive training in their use. Employees must be trained that fire extinguishers are to be used only for small fires. A back up extinguisher should be available as well. Employees should be instructed to never let a fire back them into a corner; they should always have an exit route when using a fire extinguisher.

AED

An automated external defibrillator (AED) is a device that can be used in an emergency situation when a person's heart has stopped beating (cardiac arrest). It works by delivering an electrical impulse (shock) that restarts the stopped heart. These should only be used by those that have been trained to use them in an approved first aid course. The device consists of two adhesive pads that are wired to the defibrillator. The device can assess the person's heart rhythm and recommend whether defibrillation is indicated. These pads are placed on either side of the heart on a dry chest, generally the patient's top right and lower left torso, per the equipment's directions. CPR should continue until the pads are in place. Hold CPR and press "analyze" to allow the device to analyze the rhythm and identify the indication for defibrillation. If defibrillation is indicated (in the case of ventricular fibrillation or pulseless ventricular tachycardia), the machine will announce that the pads are being charged and then instruct its user to administer the shock. Prior to administering the shock, all individuals should confirm that they are "clear" (not contacting the patient). Immediately after the shock is delivered, CPR should resume. The AED will continue to provide instructions for further rhythm analysis and shocks. Continue CPR and follow the AED's instructions until emergency responders arrive.

CPR

CPR is a technique used in emergencies by first responders to try to restart a heart that has stopped beating (heart attack). It is important that it be performed by trained personnel; however, a basic familiarity with the technique should be had by all. It involves checking to ensure there are no airway obstructions, then positioning the person's head so that the trachea is straight and the head back. Two quick breaths are given by mouth while pinching the nose closed to see if this action

142

revives the person. If not, and there is no heartbeat, 30 chest compressions are given, followed by two breaths. The cycle is repeated until another first responder relieves the person administering CPR.

BLOOD-BORNE PATHOGENS

Blood-borne pathogens are disease-causing agents that can be transmitted from one person to another by contact with the blood or bodily fluids of a person who is infected with them. Examples of blood-borne pathogens include hepatitis, human immunodeficiency virus (HIV), and Ebola virus. Employees may be at risk of infection by blood-borne pathogens while administering first aid or during an injury situation. They are a concern because the diseases that are transmitted by contact with blood or bodily fluid are serious with severe and sometimes fatal consequences. In addition, they do not have successful cures available, so if one becomes infected, it will impact the person for the rest of his or her life.

UNIVERSAL PRECAUTIONS

"Universal precautions" is a term used in the control of occupational exposure to blood-borne pathogens. The premise is that any and all blood and bodily fluids are potentially contaminated with blood-borne pathogens such as HIV or hepatitis and should, therefore, be treated as such. The universal precautions to be employed are to wear proper protective equipment when handling these items (latex gloves and eye protection) and to ensure that all surfaces contaminated with blood are properly cleaned with a bleach solution to kill any viruses that might be present. Solid waste contaminated with blood must be contained in a plastic bag to prevent any exposure to those who may be handling it.

DISPOSING OF FIRST AID MATERIALS CONTAMINATED WITH BLOOD

During the course of administering first aid, an employer will likely generate waste materials contaminated with blood. The Bloodborne Pathogen Standard defines "regulated waste" as that which is contaminated with blood that is liquid or free-flowing. This regulated waste must be closed and contained to prevent potential contamination and exposure and should be disposed of through a licensed medical waste company. However, if there are small amounts of blood on first aid materials such as gauze pads, Band-Aids, or wound dressings that do not contain free-flowing blood, these items can be placed in a plastic bag and then placed in the regular trash and disposed of with the regular solid waste.

INCIDENT COMMAND SYSTEM (ICS)

An ICS is a standardized, multi-agency, management system designed to apply to all types of hazards from small to catastrophic. The task was mandated by Homeland Security Presidential Directive 5 and is now regulated by the National Incident Management System (NIMS). OSHA rule 1910.120 mandated the implementation of an ICS for all companies that are involved with hazardous materials. FEMA (http://training.fema.gov) provides extensive training materials to help in the development of an ICS. Deployment of an ICS is required when a hazard or natural disaster has a high potential of resulting in harm to humans, facilities, or the environment. Utilization of an ICS helps ensure safety of people and cost-effective use of resources in order to effectively manage a hazard response program.

The Incident Command System is designed to manage emergency situations effectively and efficiently. It is a standardized approach to command, control, and coordination of all types of emergency response. The structure and format of the ICS is part of the National Response System codified in the National Contingency Plan; and is widely used by government agencies when responding to disasters. The ICS is under the direction of an On-Scene Coordinator. This individual acts to coordinate the involvement of various agencies and serves as a clearinghouse for information related to the incident so that those involved coordinate effectively. The ICS is organized with divisions responsible for operations, planning, logistics and finance, with additional support for safety and information gathering and dissemination.

AGENTS THAT COULD BE USED IN TERRORIST EVENTS

Terrorists could release harmful chemical or biological agents into the air or drinking water. All over the United States, reservoirs are used for drinking water and most of them are easily accessible. Certain chemicals are extremely hazardous when inhaled (cyanide or hydrogen sulfide are fatal at low concentrations). Biological agents that are harmful if released to the public include anthrax and contagious diseases like smallpox. These materials are strictly controlled and only available in research laboratories. However, if obtained, they could be released to harm the public. Therefore, emergency planning must consider steps to take if chemical or biological agents are used in a terrorist attack.

Radioactive material could be used to produce radioactive poisoning of the public. If these agents were introduced to community water supplies or in the air over a small but highly populated area it could prove lethal. Sources of nuclear or radioactive material that could be used include research laboratories, nuclear waste facilities, and hospitals. Facilities that handle radioactive materials must have strict access controls on the materials and conduct background checks on those that handle them. Explosive agents can also be used in an attack. Some common materials used to make a bomb, include ammonium nitrate fertilizer mixed with diesel fuel. However, it does take technical expertise in order to create a device that will actually detonate. Materials that could be useful in creating an explosive device are required to be reported to the Department of Homeland Security using the CSAT (Chemical Security Assessment Tool).

Organizational Communication and Training/Education

BASIC MANAGEMENT PRINCIPLES

Efficient and effective organization involves clear lines of authority and responsibility. Organizational charts are helpful to communicate 'who reports to whom'. There should be a clear job description for each job function, detailing employee responsibilities. Top down alignment in an organizational chart is critical, but it is also helpful to see cooperation between various supervisors and managers of the same level. Many aspects of occupational hygiene and safety require participation from those who have other job functions; therefore, each job description should include a section that also documents safety tasks and responsibilities. Employees should not be allowed to refuse to do tasks that are not explicitly listed in their job descriptions; they should be written broadly enough to ensure flexibility when assigning tasks.

METHODS OF COMMUNICATING

Clear communication is critical for safety. Job procedures, PPE requirements and emergency procedures should be communicated in training courses, reviewed in safety meetings, and refreshed and reinforced regularly. To help reinforce these training methods, communication aids should be created and posted in the work areas to serve as a reference and a reminder.

Job procedures – should be written in a way that communicates in words the steps needed to complete a given job safely. The procedure should also use pictures and illustrations as much as possible so that communication is visual as well as written. These can be posted at the point of use as a reference and reminder.

Personal Protective Equipment – required PPE should be listed and posted near the equipment along with a photograph or illustration for clarity.

Emergency Procedures – Emergency exit routes should be clearly indicated on facility evacuation maps that are posted in work areas. It is also helpful to have evacuation routes drawn on the floor in reflective paint. Emergency exits must be indicated with lighted signs. An emergency procedures checklist should be readily available in the work area that lists any equipment that should be de-energized during emergencies. Also, someone must be designated to ensure everyone has evacuated a given area and accounted for in the assembly area.

TYPES OF RECORDS THAT MUST BE RETAINED

Recordkeeping is one of the most important aspects of occupational hygiene and safety because it provides a basis for independent verification that compliance was achieved. It is also critical for having a properly documented record in the event of an injury. Records must be kept of initial and annual OSHA training classes to show that employees have been properly instructed regarding potential hazards of their jobs and how to protect themselves. Medical clearance records must be maintained. Industrial hygiene testing records must be retained to show that exposure levels are within acceptable limits. Routine safety inspection records must be kept to show that equipment is maintained properly and that emergency equipment is available (i.e. fire extinguishers). Employee injury documentation must include accident investigations, work status reports from the physician, and records of restricted duty offered and accepted.

MEANS OF CONFLICT RESOLUTION

There are five common methods of handling conflict. Each can be classified as either assertive or unassertive and cooperative or uncooperative.

- *Avoidance* – This occurs when the person simply avoids the situation. It is unassertive and uncooperative
- *Accommodation* – This occurs when a person simply gives in to the desires of other parties. It is unassertive and cooperative
- *Competition* – This occurs when a person demands his or her needs be met at the expense of others' needs being met. It is assertive and uncooperative
- *Collaboration* – This occurs when a person wants his or her needs met but is willing to seek solutions that would satisfy others' needs as well. It is assertive and cooperative
- *Compromise* – This occurs when a person is willing to reach a middle ground solution so that everyone's needs are met. It strikes a balance between assertiveness and unassertiveness and cooperative and uncooperative behavior

There is no absolute correct way of handling conflict. Each method serves a purpose, but some may be more effective than others.

- *Avoidance* – This is reserved for issues that are unimportant or for situations when the danger of using other methods is greater than the potential benefit
- *Accommodation* – This is used if one side is clearly right or if the issue is less important to one side than the other
- *Competition* – This is most useful in situations in which a quick decision must be made or one side simply holds more power than the other
- *Collaboration* – This is suitable when both sides have good points and it is in the company's best interest to synthesize them
- *Compromise* – This is useful in situations where both sides hold equal sway and reaching a mutually exclusive decision would be too disruptive or would consume too many resources

ADULT LEARNING THEORY

Adults come to work with a wealth of life and employment experiences. Their attitudes toward education may vary considerably. There are, however, some principles of adult learning and typical characteristics of adult learners that an instructor should consider when planning strategies for teaching:

- Practical and goal-oriented:
  o Provide overviews or summaries and examples.
  o Use collaborative discussions with problem-solving exercises.
  o Remain organized with the goal in mind.
- Self-directed:
  o Provide active involvement, asking for input.
  o Allow different options toward achieving the goal.
  o Give them responsibilities.
- Knowledgeable:
  o Show respect for their life experiences/ education.
  o Validate their knowledge and ask for feedback.
  o Relate new material to information with which they are familiar.

- Relevancy-oriented:
  - Explain how information will be applied on the job.
  - Clearly identify objectives.
- Motivated:
  - Provide certificates of professional advancement and/or continuing education credit when possible.

EFFECTIVE TEACHING TECHNIQUES FOR ADULT LEARNERS

Well-designed training courses for adults will have at least three qualities: the training will be relevant to the group, it will provide current information not already known to the participants, and it will build upon their experience. Techniques that have proven useful to promote these three qualities include using hands-on experiences or exercises as a group or in small subgroups (for example, assembling a respirator), providing opportunities for discussion that honors the participants' experience, and allowing participants to demonstrate their newly acquired knowledge in a safe and nonjudgmental environment (for example, running a mock emergency scenario after the participants learn the principles of emergency response).

TRAINING DELIVERY MEDIUMS AND TECHNOLOGIES

Safety training can be difficult and tedious, but it is critical for worker health. Classroom training is beneficial because content can be tailored to the audience and work environment. It also allows for personal interaction and hands-on training activities that enhance learning. The disadvantages include the difficulty of scheduling a class that can accommodate everybody who needs to take the class. Usually multiple times and locations must be offered. Online training classes are an attractive option because they can be completed whenever the individual has the time. However, they tend to be generic and not tailored to the audience or specific work environment. Sitting in front of a computer terminal is often boring, and it is more difficult for employees to understand and retain information delivered this way.

There are several important considerations when developing a training presentation. First, the regulatory requirements for the training class must be known. This includes what specific information must be covered and who must attend. It is also critical to take into account the level of technical knowledge, language proficiency, and previous training that those taking the class possess. Determine how long it will take to cover the material and how much time has been allotted for the class. Create an outline of the material and incorporate multimedia portions along with hands-on activities. Find ways to encourage class participation and discussion in order to promote and sustain interest. The best training classes will also include an assessment portion in order to determine whether the class has improved understanding of the topic.

CHOOSING APPROPRIATE TRAINING

A variety of training techniques should be used to teach and reinforce concepts. The best training programs use a combination of all three methods. Traditional classroom lecture-style training is useful when the topic is academic in nature. For example, it can be helpful to explain lockout/tagout regulations and procedures in a classroom setting. Demonstration training is best when the topic involves physical manipulation of an object. An example of demonstration training is teaching the use of a respirator, how to disassemble and maintain it. On-the-job training refers to training in specific tasks and occurs in the actual work environment. Written reference material and job aids should be available to reinforce the proper performance of each task. In the example of lockout/tagout above, on-the-job training should be conducted with each piece of equipment to show employees where the lockout points are, and to demonstrate proper isolation of the energy source.

TRAINING EVALUATION METHODS

There are several effective methods to evaluate the effectiveness of a training course. The most well-known and traditional method is to administer a written quiz or exam at the end of the course that covers the information presented in the course. Some types of learning are best evaluated by requiring the course participant to demonstrate a newly acquired skill to the course instructor, such as how to perform CPR or how to wear an SCBA respirator. Requiring a team of coworkers to apply newly acquired knowledge in a tabletop exercise is also an effective method of evaluating the effectiveness of a training course. An example of this type of evaluation is to require a group that has just received disaster planning training to plan for a specific disaster scenario as assigned by the instructor. What is important to remember when planning training evaluation tools is that methods other than written quizzes can be equally effective and more useful to the participants.

Evaluating the effectiveness of training is important to ensure that employees really understand the material presented. Evaluation can take several forms, but the most common are a written test, a demonstration test, and post-training observation. A written test can be multiple-choice or fill in the blanks, and can be administered as a pre- and post-test to gauge knowledge before and after training. One drawback to a written test is the possibility that employees have limited English proficiency. The test can be presented in the employee's native language or other methods used to increase understanding. A demonstration test requires the employee to perform a task in front of the evaluator, and the evaluator rates the employee on their performance. An example of this type of test is the behind-the-wheel portion of forklift training. Post-training observation is similar, but is conducted when employees are not aware they are being tested by observing them doing a task to see whether they have mastered it.

METHODS OF ASSESSING EMPLOYEE COMPETENCY

Competency (defined as possessing sufficient knowledge or skill) should be assessed to determine whether an employee requires supplemental training or resources to work safely. The following four methods can be used to assess competency:

- **Test**: the most common method, a test to evaluate knowledge of the topic is inexpensive and easy to execute. The shortcoming of testing is that it only evaluates knowledge, not ability.
- **Self-assessment**: the employee provides feedback by evaluating their own abilities. The benefit of a self-assessment is that the employee can identify areas they feel they need to improve. This method can suffer from an employee's fear of consequences if they appear substandard or provide an unrealistic assessment of their shortcomings.
- **Feedback**: the supervisor or coworkers provide feedback on the abilities of the employee based on past performance. This method suffers from the potential of bias because personal feelings can impact the truthfulness of the assessment.
- **Skills test**: the employee demonstrates their abilities in a controlled environment. This method demonstrates what the employee can do, does not bias against those who struggle with written tests, and can test the employee's ability to adapt to unusual situations. However, it can be expensive if a test laboratory must be constructed or if the observation slows the production line.

COMPETENCY-BASED TRAINING

Competency-based training is a method of safety training that requires employees to demonstrate their ability to perform the skills conveyed during training. Instead of only verifying that an individual has received the information (typically evaluated using a written test), this method relies on performance-based assessments that allow the employee to demonstrate their understanding and application of the knowledge. For example, instead of having an employee complete a written exam on the steps needed to check a respirator prior to use, the evaluator would give the employee a respirator and observe them conducting the checks while donning the respirator.

WELL-DESIGNED PRESENTATIONS

Developing effective training presentations begins with understanding the information to be conveyed, and why it needs to be taught. Is it a regulatory requirement? What are the consequences if employees do not understand the information? Next, consideration needs to be given to the needs of the audience. For example, what is the educational level, literacy level, and native language of the employees to be trained? The presentation must be tailored to their needs. For example, native Spanish speakers prefer to have training classes delivered in Spanish. Any slides used in the presentations should have plenty of visual elements and minimize wordiness. Finally, consideration should be given to developing presentations that use a variety of techniques all in the same class. There should be multimedia elements, hands-on activities, group break-out sessions, and group discussions to engage the audience and to retain interest in the topic.

Ethics and Professional Conduct

OBLIGATION TO ENSURE SAFETY INFORMATION IS UNDERSTOOD

Although it seems obvious that employees must actually understand safe work practices, there are specific OSHA regulations that require demonstration of employee understanding. Process safety management regulations require that an employer be able to demonstrate how it was verified that employees understood the material presented to them. A common way to do this is to have employees take an exam to demonstrate proficiency with the concepts. If employees do not have sufficient understanding of English to understand spoken and written communication, translated materials should be provided, and work instructions should use photos and illustrations as much as possible to communicate information. OSHA regulations on personal protective equipment require that an employee be able to demonstrate proper use of the PPE. For example, with regard to using a respirator, employees must be able to demonstrate checking the seal or fit, inspecting the equipment, putting it on properly, and maintaining it. For lockout/tagout, employees must be able to demonstrate safe removal of energy controls.

BCSP CODE OF ETHICS AND PROFESSIONAL CONDUCT

The Board of Certified Safety Professionals (BCSP) has established a code of ethics and professional conduct that must be followed by individuals who are awarded certificates by this organization. The first two standards of this code promote the need for certificate holders to support and promote the integrity, esteem, and influence of the safety occupation. The code prioritizes human safety and health as the top concern in any scenario. Additional focus should also be given to environmental safety and the protection of property. Each of these priorities can be promoted by safety professionals in warning people of hazards and risks. These standards also include the promotion of honest and fair behavior toward all individuals and organizations and the avoidance of any behavior that would dishonor the esteem or reputation of the safety profession.

Standard 1 focuses on the primary responsibility of a safety professional to protect the safety and health of humans. A specific component of this responsibility is the need to notify appropriate personnel, management, and agencies regarding hazardous or potentially hazardous situations. An example might be a scenario in which a safety professional is analyzing company records of employee exposures to potentially hazardous materials on a consultant basis. The safety professional discovers a calculation mistake in transferring readings from a personal monitor into a formula that calculates the daily exposure rate. This mistake has resulted in underestimating the exposure rate by as much as 50%. The safety professional immediately notes these findings in an urgent communication to the company. He then follows up with the company on correcting the calculation errors immediately for present and future employees and determining actions to take for employees that might have already received hazardous levels of exposure.

Standard 2 specifically deals with the safety professional's character. The safety professional should "be honest, fair, and impartial; act with responsibility and integrity…" The safety professional has to balance the interests of all involved parties and represent the profession in all business dealings.

Standard 3 focuses on appropriate public statements and contact. This standard notes that honesty and objectivity are required in all communications and statements. Safety professionals should only make statements related to areas or situations about which they have direct expertise.

Standard 4 focuses on the professional status and actions of safety professionals. A safety professional should only engage in projects or activities for which they are highly qualified in terms of knowledge, training, and experience. Additionally, ongoing education and professional advancement activities should be pursued by all safety professionals to maintain and improve knowledge and skill level, as well as to maintain certification. The BCSP supports annual conferences that enable safety professionals to receive valuable training and education while accumulating points required to keep their certification current.

Standard 5 focuses on integrity and honesty in the presentation of professional qualifications. This includes areas such as education, degrees, certification, experience, and achievements. Not only must safety professionals be careful to clearly and honestly state all qualifications, but any exaggeration or misrepresentation by omission must also be avoided. When applying for jobs, providing references, or testifying in court, a safety professional must not lie about their employment history, professional relationships, or professional qualifications and experience. A safety professional with knowledge about violations of this standard should report the information to the BCSP.

Standard 6 specifies that the OHST should avoid all conflicts of interest in order to maintain the integrity of their profession. Section 7 focuses on avoiding discrimination and bias. It is specifically noted that OHST's must not discriminate or demonstrate bias based on gender, age, race, ethnicity, country of origin, sexual orientation, or disability. These areas are also regulated by local, state, and federal agencies enforcing Civil Right and other related anti-discrimination legislation. Section 8 of this code promotes the need for OHST's to be involved in community and civic events and use their professional qualifications to promote safety within their own community. Examples of this include instructing public safety personnel in handling hazardous materials, teaching public safety classes in areas of fire prevention, home safety, and accident prevention. OHST's can work cooperatively with organizations and agencies already working in the community such as the Red Cross, fire departments, and police departments.

The impartiality principle of the Board of Certified Safety Professionals (BCSP) Code of Ethics holds that:

An Occupational Hygiene and Safety Technician (OHST) should adhere to the impartiality principle in all interactions and engage the advice and support of supervisors in determining appropriate actions. One area of concern is to avoid conflicts of interest or promoting oneself beyond actual expertise or competence. For example, if asked to testify in a lawsuit that revolves around an incident involving a former employee of a company affiliated with the OHST's employer, the OHST should defer to avoid conflict of interest. Another example would be a OHST who is asked to testify to the appropriateness of safety procedures related to radioactive materials. Although the OHST received general instruction in this area in a course, he has no direct experience. He should decline to avoid presenting himself as an expert in that area.

The Code of Ethics and Professional Conduct for safety professionals notes that the primary responsibility of a safety professional is to safeguard the health and safety of humans, as well as to provide for the safety of the environment and property. In a typical construction site, numerous organizations, individuals, and entities are working jointly to complete the project. Ultimately, each organization or company bears responsibility for making sure its workers are well trained and have a safe work environment. A main function in ensuring a safe worksite is to include safety stipulations in the contracts of all involved individuals or organizations.

An OHST must earn at least 25 points every five-year period, based on continuing education and professional development in order to retain their certificate.

PROTECTING CONFIDENTIAL INFORMATION

Employers are not entitled to all the health and safety information of employees. There are legal privacy protections under the Health Insurance Portability and Accountability Act (HIPAA) that protects employee's health information if it is not connected to a work-related injury, request for sick leave, or provision of health insurance. Health information provided to the employer must be authorized by the employee. Employers are authorized to receive work readiness health information for employees that have work-related injuries. These are not actual medical records but are the physician's assessment of an employee's work restrictions or prognosis. Alcohol and substance abuse records are not considered occupational health records. There are other health-related records employers are obligated to retain. For example, records of employee exposures to toxic materials must be retained for thirty years. This includes industrial hygiene monitoring records and the results of any biological monitoring such as blood lead levels or cadmium in urine levels. Results of audiometry must be similarly retained. The purpose of this requirement is that certain adverse exposure outcomes may take years to manifest (such as hearing loss or cancer) and exposure records need to be available in case there is a possibility that the problem is work-related.

TRADE SECRETS

A trade secret is information specific to a business or operation that has inherent economic value that a competitor could use to his advantage. Trade secrets include processes, customer lists and relationships, and designs. To prove that something is a trade secret, companies must demonstrate the extent to which the information has been protected and the extent to which people inside the business know the information. For example, a trade secret is not normally known by all employees, but only those that have the need to know the information. Companies must also demonstrate the measures taken to protect the information; for example, storing the data on computer systems that cannot be accessed without authorized passwords. Trade secrets must also be of demonstrable value to others and, therefore, worth protecting. Well-known examples of trade secrets include the formula for Coca-Cola or the algorithm Google uses in its search engine.

OHST Practice Test

Want to take this practice test in an online interactive format?
Check out the online resources page, which includes interactive practice
questions and much more: **mometrix.com/resources719/ohst**

1. Which of the following is generally true with regard to worksite safety inspections?

    a. Unbiased inspections are best conducted by personnel who only have a generalist's knowledge of the subject area being inspected.
    b. The most useful findings come from scheduled inspections.
    c. Inspections, by design, should always be generically oriented in nature.
    d. Inspectors are independent entities who do not have a direct affiliation with the organization or entity undergoing inspection.

2. A robust incident reporting system typically includes which of the following facets?

    a. Mechanisms for filing "lessons learned"
    b. Remote electronic access capabilities in the field
    c. Clear direction on how to differentiate and properly distinguish among incident severity categories
    d. Established processes for commencing worker compensation claims

3. Which of the following is a major advantage that is characteristic of undergoing an external versus internal audit?

    a. Benchmarking of audit findings against those of competitors
    b. Higher levels of subsequent managerial engagement in response to findings
    c. More rapid initiation of corrective actions in response to discovered findings
    d. Direct national certification opportunities (e.g., International Organization for Standardization [ISO] and ANSI) are more readily available via external audit corrective action measures

4. Which of the following is often associated with frostbite of the fingers or toes?

    a. Absence of pain
    b. Fibromyalgia
    c. Chilblains
    d. Localized capillary damage to the hands and feet from high blood pressure

5. Besides lead, which of the following is also typically utilized as a robust shielding material for protection against gamma or X-ray radiation?

    a. Aluminum
    b. Water
    c. Lithium
    d. Beryllium

6. Which of the following is often a typical means by which hazards can arise during the conduct of maintenance activities?

    a. Maintenance procedures are being followed in too literal of a fashion.
    b. Manufacturer recommendations are regularly superseding internally driven mandates.
    c. Maintenance schedules are not adhered to.
    d. Over-allocation of resources is selected for maintenance items.

7. The tangent of angle ∠ABC (note: drawing is not to scale) is equal to:

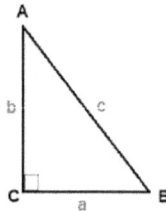

    a. b/a
    b. c/b
    c. a/b
    d. a/c

8. Which of the following is NOT a widely employed method used in industry for reducing hazardous noise levels?

    a. Using sound-absorbent materials in building construction
    b. Decreasing vibrational frequencies
    c. Employing white-noise background sources for dilution
    d. Decreasing flow rates

9. What type of glove material is widely used for protecting the hands against welding sparks?

    a. Neoprene
    b. Polyester
    c. Leather
    d. Polyethylene

10. What is the statistical median of the following data set (6, 13, 15, 15, 18, 24, 28, 33, 51, and 66)?

    a. 26.9
    b. 18 and 24
    c. 21
    d. 36

11. What is typically regarded as the MOST difficult challenge associated with the generation of a cost-benefit analysis?

    a. The performance of associated cost-benefit analysis risk assessments
    b. Determining how much a human-life is "worth" from a financial perspective
    c. Accurately determining potential long-term cost savings of a proposed safety enhancement
    d. Substantiating design-basis criteria

12. Which of the following project management tools can be effectively used for comprehensively illustrating a project schedule?

    a. GANTT chart
    b. Work breakdown structure (WBS)
    c. Scope of work (SOW)
    d. Project plan

13. Which of the following tenets is typically NOT true in regard to the concept of continual improvement?

    a. An organization should not seek perfection as the ultimate goal for achievement.
    b. Performance improvement should be sought at a variety of paces, depending on the circumstances.
    c. Large-scale improvement initiatives as opposed to incremental improvements should ultimately be sought.
    d. Lessons-learned programs should be integrated with continual improvement programs.

14. Which of the following four-step models is of chief importance and highly utilized within occupational safety and health programs?

    a. Stop-observe-respond-report
    b. Plan-do-check-act
    c. Appraise-respond-evaluate-learn
    d. Educate-implement-adjust-document

15. Which of the following would NOT be considered a benefit of commencing an accident investigation as soon as possible?

    a. The sooner the causes are found, the sooner appropriate culpability can be assigned.
    b. Future accident costs can ultimately be reduced via the prompt attainment of accident root causes.
    c. A rapidly commenced investigation sends a message of robust corporate engagement.
    d. Rapid investigations help ensure that the incident is still fresh in the minds of those from whom information is being gathered.

16. Which of the following is a typically implemented protocol for protecting workers from blood-borne pathogens?

    a. Washing one's hands after removing protective glove wear
    b. Regular employee health screenings and medical monitoring
    c. Requiring infectious personnel to wear additional personal protective equipment (PPE)
    d. Requesting that infectious personnel provide disclosure

17. Which of the following is one of Heinrich's 10 Axioms of Workplace Safety?

    a. Knowing why people work unsafely does not directly initiate appropriate corrective measures.
    b. Accident prevention strategies usually function independently of production and quality strategies.
    c. Most accidents are the result of unsafe worker behavior.
    d. Senior management should retain a degree of independence and separation from the realm of workplace safety.

18. According to the Errors in Management Systems theory (developed by Juran and Deming), approximately what percentage of workplace errors are usually the result of poor management procedures and/or processes?
   a. 35%
   b. 50%
   c. 70%
   d. 85%

19. If a work area has dimensions of 30 ft x 18 ft x 8 ft, what is the shortest amount of time it could potentially take for the entire supply of air in the room to (hypothetically) be completely exchanged via an air-exchanger HVAC system that operates at a rate of 60 cfm?
   a. 1.2 hrs
   b. 2.2 hrs
   c. 2.9 hrs
   d. 3.4 hrs

20. Which of the following is a type of hearing hazard that can result from exposure to excessively loud noises?
   a. Variance in equilibrium
   b. Shifts in threshold
   c. Eustachianary fibrillation
   d. Celiac fibromyalgia

21. Which of the following machine components typically entails the hazard of potential nip points?
   a. Bushings
   b. Guards
   c. Gears
   d. Actuators

22. Which of the following is typically considered one of the fundamental principles of ergonomics?
   a. Workforce comfort should be assessed as an aggregate entity.
   b. Output should never trump common sense.
   c. Whenever possible, the job should be changed and not the worker.
   d. A workstation should always be a work in progress.

23. Which of the following is considered a robust physical control against electrical hazards?
   a. Utilizing inductors for maintaining adequate grounding
   b. Use of nonconductive gels during high-voltage maintenance activities
   c. Use of impedance-relay devices for diverting current
   d. Utilizing wires that are not excessively long

24. Which of the following is NOT typically employed as a control strategy for protecting against confined-space hazards?
   a. Ensuring adequate fire-suppression equipment is available
   b. Use of a buddy system
   c. Evaluating potential hazards of the space immediately after entry
   d. Ensuring adequate ventilation is at hand

25. Which of the following is generally NOT true regarding chemical irritants?
    a. The mucus membranes are often easily affected by these agents.
    b. Permanent tissue damage often occurs as a result of exposure.
    c. Chemical irritants can cause dermatitis.
    d. Hair spray is an example of a chemical irritant.

26. Which of the following is generally true regarding biohazards?
    a. Biohazards can be either animal or plant based.
    b. Biohazards are not fungal based.
    c. Biohazards, by definition, are not allergenic in nature.
    d. Biohazards are usually transmitted through the air.

27. In regard to worker injury and incident statistics, (Number of OSHA recordable injuries x 200,000) ÷ (total hours worked) is used to calculate which of the following metrics?
    a. Lost time incident rate (LTIR)
    b. Days away from work rate (DAWR)
    c. Days away, restricted duty, or transfer (DART) rate
    d. Total recordable incident rate (TRIR)

28. Which of the following is a regularly employed tactic for combating sick office syndrome?
    a. Maintaining low building humidity levels
    b. Implementing isolation areas for sick personnel to exclusively conduct work
    c. Replacing furniture
    d. Having floors tiled instead of carpeted

29. Which of the following is an established principle used for the implementation of proper workstation configurations?
    a. Usage economics
    b. Usage sharing
    c. Usage parametrization
    d. Usage sequence

30. Which of the following is generally true with regard to building evacuation plans?
    a. Plans should include fire extinguishing protocols.
    b. Plans should specify locations of indoor shelter-in-place areas.
    c. Plans should include procedures on how to activate emergency response teams in tandem with an evacuation.
    d. Plans should be designed so that personnel (still) know where to exit during a darkness blackout.

31. Which of the following is generally true of recirculated-air system operational requirements?
    a. Cleaning systems must have secondary and tertiary filtration modules that maintain efficiencies of at least 90% and 75%, respectively, of the primary module's efficiency.
    b. Contaminated air must be contained indoors in the event of an incident.
    c. Recirculated air must undergo regular sampling and evaluation to verify that cleaning systems are correctly functioning.
    d. Cleaning systems must have audio warning indicators of at least 80 dB (at 3 feet) to advise personnel of potential issues.

32. Which of the following is an example of an electrical-switching device that is typically used in the workplace for reducing electrical hazards?

a. Modulators
b. Interlocks
c. Transducers
d. Phase actuators

33. Lower-back injuries typically comprise approximately what percentage of worker compensation claims across all industries?

a. 5%
b. 15%
c. 25%
d. 40%

34. Which of the following sets of worker behavioral dynamics often results from increased levels of industrial automation (i.e., less manpower) within a workplace setting?

a. Normlessness-powerlessness-mindlessness
b. Paranoia-ineffectiveness-indifference
c. Objectivity-irrelevance-extrication
d. Antagonism-resignation-helplessness

35. Which of the following is a typical "standardized" approach or process used in industry for asbestos abatement?

a. Entrenchment
b. Restoration
c. Replacement
d. Encapsulation

36. Which of the following is a typical benefit associated with the use of ventilation systems?

a. They help reduce the buildup of carbon dioxide.
b. They help facilitate the conversion of ozone into free oxygen.
c. They help keep vapor concentrations at ignitable thresholds.
d. They help to balance out equilibrium losses that often occur during atmospheric inversions.

37. What should be the first step implemented in the development of a robust facility emergency plan?

a. Submitting a plan license application request to OSHA and FEMA
b. Assembling a plan team from a variety of organizational functions and disciplines
c. Creating a disaster-response draft procedure
d. Constructing a general plan mission statement for approval by the facility general manager

38. What is typically regarded as the MOST important reason for conducting a workplace safety analysis?

a. To help avoid accidents by determining what hazards exist and what controls are required to avoid them
b. To provide higher ROIs over the long term due to lower worker compensation premiums
c. Because it is an OSHA requirement per 29 CFR 1926.70
d. To be able to prequalify for VPP-Star status

39. What is typically regarded as a most effective method or model for conducting a root-cause analysis?

- a. The Multiple-Tier method
- b. The Failure Sequence and Effects model
- c. The Five-Why method
- d. The Six Sigma Cause and Effect model

40. Which of the following materials acts as a good electrical insulator?

- a. Copper
- b. Mercury
- c. Oil
- d. Carbon

41. Electrical fires often occur due to electrical _____ or poor _____.

- a. surges/impedance
- b. shorts/connections
- c. flux/insulation
- d. bonding/voltage regulation

42. What is the overall calculated annual risk of an accident event that has a frequency of 0.0005 per year and an associated consequence of 1.4 fatalities?

- a. 1.4 fatalities per year
- b. 0.0005 fatalities per year
- c. 0.00070 fatalities per year
- d. 0.00036 fatalities per year

43. A histogram most closely resembles which of the following in appearance?

- a. Scatterplot
- b. Critical-path trend plot
- c. Step-function plot
- d. Bar graph

44. Which of the following cost-benefit analysis outcomes depicts a worst-case project choice?

- a. $\{ \sum \$Benefits / \sum \$Costs \} = 1$
- b. $\{ \sum \$Benefits / \sum \$Costs \} > 1$
- c. $\{ \sum \$Benefits / \sum \$Costs \} < 1$
- d. $\{ \sum \$Benefits / \sum \$Costs \} = 0$

45. Which of the following is true with regard to statistical correlation coefficients?

- a. A coefficient of –1 reflects a neutral correlation between two variables.
- b. A coefficient of 0 reflects a very strong correlation between two variables.
- c. They depict how robust the functional relationship is between a linear regression equation's primary variable and beta value.
- d. Determining these values can serve as a robust indicator as to whether a given equation for a best-fit line is accurate.

46. **Which of the following is typically evaluated within the domain of accident prevention?**
    a. Accident liabilities
    b. Accident responsibilities
    c. Accident financial impacts
    d. Accident cycles

47. **If a horizontal section of ground needs to exert a force of 12.5 newtons (N) to support an object, what is the mass of the object?**
    a. 17.9 pounds
    b. 1.28 kilograms
    c. 0.047 pounds
    d. 0.61 kilograms

48. **A type-A-rated fire extinguisher is effective against which type of fire?**
    a. Electrical equipment
    b. Laboratory chemicals
    c. Trash, wood, or paper
    d. Flammable liquids

49. **Which of the following radiation types are anti-contamination / respirator tandems MOST effective at protecting workers against?**
    a. Alpha
    b. Neutron
    c. Gamma
    d. Microwave

50. **In EPA-space, the term TSCA is an acronym for which of the following?**
    a. Treat-Stabilize-Control-Administer
    b. Teratogenic Separation Cooperative Amendment
    c. Transportation of Surplus Contaminated Actinides
    d. Toxic Substances Control Act

51. **Which of the following would be considered the LEAST dangerous to overall human health?**
    a. 1 M nitric acid
    b. 2 M hydrochloric acid
    c. 3 M acetic acid
    d. 4 M hydrofluoric acid

52. **Which of the following four elements is part of the fire tetrahedron?**
    a. Combustible material
    b. Air
    c. Smoke
    d. Chain reaction

53. In regard to chemical hazard exposure limits, which of the following is an established parametric acronym implemented and exercised by the American Conference of Governmental Industrial Hygienists (ACGIH)?

    a. STEL
    b. MAL
    c. CHLA
    d. DELA

54. The Occupational Safety and Health Act mandates that employers provide _____ for/to their employees.

    a. safety and health training
    b. worker compensation benefits
    c. health insurance options
    d. workplace safety inspections

55. Which government agency should be immediately notified (first) in the event of any accidental release of hazardous materials during their transportation?

    a. US Federal Emergency Management Agency (FEMA)
    b. US Department of Transportation (DOT)
    c. US National Transportation Safety Board (NTSB)
    d. US Department of Homeland Security (DHS)

56. For the six variables conventionally applied (H-V-D-F-A-C) in determining recommended weight limits, what does the D denote?

    a. Horizontal travel distance
    b. Fixed distance
    c. Degree of rotational freedom
    d. Vertical travel distance

57. Which of the following is typically considered a natural-based hazard that can often lead to fires and/or explosions?

    a. High outdoor temperature indexes
    b. Floods
    c. Solar flares
    d. High winds

58. Which pathway entrance into the body is typically most hazardous for a potential intake or uptake of radon?

    a. Inhalation
    b. Absorption
    c. Ingestion
    d. Osmosis

59. Which of the following forms of environmental media typically requires a corporate entity to attain a state regulatory permit?

    a. Soil or sediment translocation
    b. Sanitary or sewer waste
    c. Storm water runoff
    d. Borehole thermal emissions

60. **When a chemical reaction occurs between an acid and a base, water and what other material class is generally produced?**
    a. Hydrogen
    b. Salt
    c. Hydroxyl
    d. Chelate

61. **A fitness-for-duty assessment, conducted by employers, is often used to determine whether a candidate or present employee is (or is not) able to perform requisite job duties because of physical or _____ limitations.**
    a. training
    b. competency
    c. psychological
    d. educational

62. **What aspect of fire-related emergencies is typically responsible for the most fatalities?**
    a. Heat-induced trauma
    b. Shock
    c. Smoke inhalation
    d. Damage to tissues

63. **Which of the following is typically associated with excessive exposures to vibrating machinery?**
    a. Muscular dystrophy
    b. Fibromyalgia
    c. Hypoxia
    d. White-finger syndrome

64. **What is an endeavor to uncover and reduce hazards that may be at hand for product or system users as well as to those who are accountable for their maintenance conventionally known as?**
    a. Preliminary hazard analysis
    b. Occupational health hazard assessment
    c. Documented safety analysis
    d. Technical safety requirement evaluation

65. **A Hazard and Operability Study (HAZOP) is a regimented and methodical evaluation of a planned or existing undertaking or process in an attempt to identify and assess potential issues that may ultimately culminate in risks to _____.**
    a. workers, equipment, and/or operational efficiencies
    b. operational revenues
    c. design safety bases
    d. the environment

66. **What is typically deemed as a vital component of workstation proper seating posture?**
    a. Keeping one's chin elevated as high as comfortably possible
    b. Keeping the forearms parallel to the floor
    c. Maintaining a computer screen distance of at least 30 inches for a 20/20 vision line of sight
    d. Positioning both feet with the toes higher than the heels

67. Which of the following materials is conventionally utilized as a fire suppressant?

    a. Lithium sulfide
    b. Calcium triphosphate
    c. Ozone
    d. Potassium bicarbonate

68. The following series of force equations characterizes a static hoist apparatus used in the workplace for a given task:

$$2x_1 + x_2 - 4x_3 = 6 \ N$$
$$5y_1 = 3.5 \ N$$
$$x_3 = 2y_1$$

What is the calculated force of x_2 given that $x_1 \neq 0$?

    a. 2.250 newtons
    b. 5.167 newtons
    c. 14.429 newtons
    d. cannot be determined from the information provided

69. OSHA's General Duty Clause, Section 5(a)(1) covers (and enforces) the broad topic of worker _____.

    a. confined space requirements
    b. ergonomics
    c. personal protective equipment (PPE)
    d. medical monitoring

70. There are presently five (5) separate classes of fire extinguisher technologies available in modern-day industry that are designed to handle different types of fires. What are the five alpha-based codes that denote these classes?

    a. A-B-C-F-X
    b. A-B-C-D-Z
    c. A-B-C-D-K
    d. A-B-C-AA-O

71. Per EPA guidelines, which of the following is conventionally designated as a vital element of a robust environmental management system (EMS)?

    a. Maintaining internal auditor environmental-related competencies
    b. Regularly reassessing EMS fiscal (budgetary) requirements
    c. Providing in-house International Organization for Standardization (ISO) and ANSI environmental certification mechanisms
    d. Maintaining in-house environmental databases

72. An ex-employee is looking to pursue legal action against his or her company for alleged wrongdoing. The company, in turn, is planning on defending itself based upon the fellow-servant rule. Which of the following grievance subject areas is the employee pursuing legal action for?

    a. Wrongful termination
    b. On-the-job injury
    c. Racial discrimination
    d. Sexual harassment

73. Which of the following is a typical analytical endeavor or product often rendered via the National Environmental Policy Act (NEPA) of 1969?

a. Documented Safety Analysis (DSA)
b. Environmental Impact Statement (EIS)
c. Environmental Specification Basis Assessment (ESBA)
d. Annual Effluent Release Evaluation (AERE)

74. If a storage shelf has a weight-limit capacity of 200 pounds and a safe utilization surface area of 30 feet^2, how many cube-shaped 27 feet^3 boxes, with each weighing 25 pounds, can be safely stored on the shelf (note: no stacking of boxes is permitted)?

a. 3
b. 6
c. 9
d. 12

75. What is a typical net efficiency (and associated AMAD) for a filtration system to be normally categorized as a high-efficiency particulate arrestance (HEPA)?

a. 99.0%; > 10 μm diameter
b. 99.9%; > 5 μm diameter
c. 99.97%; > 3 μm diameter
d. 99.99%; > 1 μm diameter

76. The International Organization for Standardization (ISO) 9000 Standard is the MOST widely utilized guidance system in the United States for employing which of the following programs?

a. Safety management
b. Environmental management
c. Quality management and assurance
d. Work control

77. Within the realms of environmental management and the US Clean Air Act, what does the acronym RACT conventionally denote?

a. Radon airborne contaminant test
b. Resuspended atmospheric contaminant total
c. Reasonably available control technology
d. Retrofitted abatement cleansing tool

78. What device is commonly used in industrial settings to measure potentially hazardous noise levels?

a. An acoustics meter
b. A noise dosimeter
c. An audiometer
d. A gain-differential inductance meter

79. What designates what a recovery coordinator who ultimately decides what recovery actions need to be taken and assigns responsibilities for achieving such actions should do?

a. Disaster recovery plan
b. FEMA assessment action plan
c. Disaster response charter
d. Contingency recovery procedure

80. Which of the following is usually designated as a key aspect or factor when designing an enhanced ergonomic environment for older or aging workers?

a. Implementation of leverage devices
b. Use of large computer display terminals
c. Providing pneumatic-powered tools
d. Accommodating posture changes or deterioration

81. The primary EPA legislative vehicle that enforces overall standards for potable water quality is which of the following?

a. The Federal Clean Water Quality Act
b. The Comprehensive Environmental Response, Compensation, and Liability Act
c. The Potable Water Quality Act
d. The Safe Drinking Water Act

82. A company is developing a new pharmaceutical product to help counteract the effects of mercury poisoning. Before it comes to market, however, the company must first seek approval by which of the following US government agencies?

a. US Department of Health and Human Services (DHHS)
b. US National Institute for Drug Abuse (NIDA)
c. US Consumer Product Safety Commission (CPSC)
d. US Food and Drug Administration (FDA)

83. Which of the following is a typical parameter on a crane load chart for calculating safe load limits?

a. Boom angle
b. Load deviation
c. Outrigger length
d. Outrigger angle

84. Which of the following sets of colors is associated with the NFPA 704 Diamond System for the labeling of hazardous materials?

a. Magenta, green, black, gold
b. Blue, green, orange, white
c. Red, yellow, green, black
d. Yellow, blue, red, white

85. Which of the following is NOT inclusive of the OSHA Classification System for Occupational Illnesses and Conditions?

a. Respiratory-related disorders or conditions
b. Radiation-related disorders or conditions
c. Skin-related disorders or conditions
d. Blunt trauma-related disorders or conditions

86. Which of the following US federal agencies is responsible for distributing statistical information pertaining to job-related injuries and illnesses?

    a. US Occupational Safety and Health Administration
    b. US Department of Health and Human Services
    c. US Bureau of Labor Statistics
    d. US National Institute of Occupational Safety and Health

87. Per the US Nuclear Regulatory Commission's mandated annual worker dose limit of 5 rem (10 CFR 20), what percent of this limit would a worker receive if he or she were exposed to an average daily 2 millirem dose (for an 8-hour workday) over a 2,000-hour work year?

    a. 1%
    b. 10%
    c. 50%
    d. Greater than >100%

88. The _____ of activities in a project plan, which (all) must be completed on time for a given project (as a whole) to be completed on time is known as the project's critical path.

    a. full extent
    b. backlog
    c. shortest sequence
    d. longest sequence

89. Which of the following is typically true with regard to the scope of a job safety analysis (JSA)?

    a. A JSA usually does not include safety recommendations.
    b. A JSA is normally used as a precursor tool for an FMEA.
    c. A JSA outlines traceability requirements associated with a given task.
    d. A JSA is actually a "procedure" for integrating safety principles with job practices.

90. Which of the following is generally true regarding industrial hand tool design?

    a. The design should always have a top-heavy center of gravity.
    b. The design should always have the handle's center of gravity properly aligned with the center of the hand while being held.
    c. The design should always have a bottom-heavy center of gravity.
    d. Their design should never include any metallic (conducting) material in the handle or grip.

91. Which of the following liquids is considered, by far, the MOST flammable?

    a. Paraffin oil
    b. Nitromethane
    c. Dimethyl ether
    d. Biodiesel

92. Which of the following is usually responsible for initiating the MOST workplace fires?

    a. Volatile materials
    b. Arson
    c. Procedural errors
    d. Inferior electrical systems and/or poor connections

93. Which US industry is responsible for the highest frequency of fire- and explosion-related deaths?

a. Explosive ordnance fabrication
b. Mining
c. Textiles
d. Fossil fuels

94. Which of the following isotopes of hydrogen is radioactive?

a. Protium
b. Tritium
c. Deuterium
d. Heavy water

95. A back belt is a device used in the workplace for reducing the forces on the spinal column during lifting tasks via increased _____, the stimulation of core muscles and the stiffening or immobilizing of the spine.

a. Quadriceps utilization
b. Dorsal leverage
c. Abdominal pressure
d. Cervical expansion

96. Which of the following strategies is a recommended tenet from the National Institute of Occupational Safety and Health (NIOSH) for implementing an effective ergonomics program?

a. Worker interviews
b. Identifying controls
c. Repetitive-strain injury metric tracking
d. Post-diagnosis intervention

97. Which of the following is a typical symptom associated with carpal tunnel syndrome?

a. Shoulder stiffness
b. Numbness in the index finger
c. Tingling in the pinky finger
d. Swelling of the thumb

98. Which of the following classifications is often utilized for categorizing deficiencies noted during an internal or external audit?

a. Violations
b. Conditions adverse to quality
c. "Lessons learned"
d. Near misses

99. What is the recommended upper weight or force limit of an object that is to be horizontally pushed or pulled from a seated position?

a. 29-pound force
b. 33-pound force
c. 37-pound force
d. 41-pound force

100. Which of the following is a regularly utilized or measured parameter when characterizing soil quality?

    a. Aquifer flux rate
    b. Coefficient of aridity
    c. Vadosity
    d. Conductivity

101. Which of the following mitigation technologies is known to effectively eradicate biological contaminants in water?

    a. Ultraviolet light
    b. Charcoal filters
    c. Electrolysis
    d. Enzymatic reduction

102. Which of the following is considered a significant factor in determining the outcome of a potential electrocution event?

    a. The level of electrical inductance entering the body
    b. The quantity of grounded, electrically impedant material located at the exposure site
    c. The total amount of time an electrical exposure occurs
    d. How much conducting material the potential victim is wearing on his or her person

103. What is/are required under OSHA regulation 29 CFR 1910.95 (Occupational Noise Exposure) where workers may be regularly exposed to noise levels in excess of an 8-hour time-weighted average of 85 decibels (dB)?

    a. Earplugs and earmuffs
    b. Sound barriers
    c. A noise-hazard control program
    d. Semiannual auditory monitoring

104. Per 29 CFR 1910.1001, over a/an _____ time period, a worker may not be exposed to an average asbestos fiber concentration greater than 0.1 fiber per centimeter^3 of air.

    a. 1-hour
    b. 4-hour
    c. 8-hour
    d. 40-hour

105. Which of the following is specified as a hazardous waste material attribute to which the US Environmental Protection Agency extends a designated waste code (number), as per 40 CFR 261, Subpart C?

    a. Mutagenicity (#D003–#D043)
    b. Corrosivity (#D002)
    c. Teratogenicity (#D044–#D051)
    d. Volatility (#D001)

106. The formula Load Weight ÷ Recommended Weight Limit is otherwise known as which of the following?

a. Weight index
b. Lifting index
c. Leverage limit
d. Inertial pivot

107. What part of the body does a body harness typically distribute a significant amount of fall-arrest force to?

a. Bottoms of the feet
b. Thighs
c. Lower back
d. Forearms

108. The quantity of weight that healthy workers could lift for up to 8 hours without causing injuries is most accurately defined as which of the following?

a. Recommended weight limit (RWL)
b. Time-weighted-average load limit (TWALL)
c. Load weight (LW)
d. Lifting mass index (LMI)

109. The Heinrich incident-to-injury ratio model states that for every 1,000 accidents, approximately _____ will likely result in no injuries, _____ will likely cause minor injuries, and _____ will likely cause(s) major injuries.

a. 750, 225, 25
b. 833, 150, 17
c. 875, 120, 5
d. 909, 88, 3

110. The following formula [(Number of Recordable Injuries per year x 200,000) ÷ (Total Hours Worked)] depicts which of the following?

a. Recordable injury rate (RIR)
b. Total case incident rate (TCIR)
c. Days away, restricted, or transfer rate (DART)
d. OSHA 300-log reportable rate

111. Fall incidents usually account for the highest fatality rates in which of the following industries?

a. Manufacturing and processing
b. Construction
c. Transportation
d. Oil and gas

112. An electrical exposure with an associated current of 0.2 amperes would usually be expected to result in which of the following?

a. Shock
b. Unconsciousness
c. Coma
d. Death

113. The ring test is a common test used for inspecting for cracks or anomalies in which of the following industrial mechanisms?

    a. Lathe
    b. Miter saw
    c. Grinding wheel
    d. Drill press

114. An employer is ultimately responsible for ensuring that only what kind of hand and power tools are utilized on a job site?

    a. ANSI qualified
    b. Well maintained and operable
    c. QA inspected
    d. ASME certified

115. Under current laws for worker compensation, which of the following is categorized as a potential injury category?

    a. Precedential
    b. Partial
    c. Reciprocal
    d. Lateral

116. Heat stroke is typically categorized by which of the following occurrences?

    A. When most of the body's skin turns pinkish-red, particularly in the extremities
    b. When the body's temperature regulation system fails and sweating becomes inadequate
    c. When dry heaving occurs
    d. When the body's core temperature reaches at least 105.5°F

117. The Plan Do Check Act model is typically considered the cornerstone for which of the following?

    a. ANSI Z-400 Health and Safety Management System
    b. OSHA 29 CFR 1910, Subpart A, Industrial Safety Credo
    c. ISO 14001 Environmental Management System
    d. ASTM 5000X Quality Management System

118. Which of the following scenarios is indicative of a hazardous atmospheric environment?

    a. An atmospheric carbon dioxide concentration level of 500 ppm
    b. An atmospheric oxygen concentration of 23%
    c. An atmospheric oxygen concentration of 20%
    d. A flammable gas that exists at a concentration of 50% of its LFL

119. Per OSHA's 29 CFR 1904.33 (Recordkeeping Standard), how long must a document such as an OSHA Form 301 be retained?

    a. Five years following the end of the calendar year that the record covers
    b. Three years following the end of the calendar year that the record covers
    c. One year following the end of the calendar year that the record covers
    d. Seven years following the end of the calendar year that the record covers

120. Proactively identifying and responding to risk before an accident occurs is the overarching goal of which of the following?

  a. The OHSAS 18000 series of occupational health and safety management system standards
  b. The ISO 9001 Quality Management System
  c. NIOSH Guidance 961-A: Workplace Accident Prevention
  d. ANSI Standard 4882: Probabilistic Risk Assessment

121. A cut-off wheel that has a diameter of 9 inches can cut a material with which maximum thickness?

  a. 1/2 inch
  b. 1/4 inch
  c. 3/4 inch
  d. 1/8 inch

122. Per OSHA 29 CFR 1910.1025, if the permissible exposure limit (PEL) for lead (Pb) is 50 micrograms per cubic meter of air, averaged over an 8-hour period, what would MOST likely be the recommended associated action level?

  a. 30 micrograms per cubic meter of air averaged over 8 hours
  b. 50 micrograms per cubic meter of air averaged over 8 hours
  c. 500 micrograms per cubic meter of air averaged over 8 hours
  d. 0.5 microgram per cubic meter of air averaged over 8 hours

123. A tagout process must be implemented when an energy-isolation device is not able to be locked out. Which of the following is a typical requirement associated with the tagout process?

  a. Tags must be red, magenta, or black in color.
  b. Tags must always be suspended in at least one location by a metallic clip.
  c. Tags must display either the term "High-Energy Hazard" or "Electrical Hazard" (as applicable) on its outward-facing side.
  d. Tags must be normalized to a consistent shape and size.

124. Standards for _____ are regularly set by the American National Standards Institute.

  a. chemical exposure limits
  b. SI units
  c. protective eyewear
  d. asbestos abatement protocols

125. If an employee death occurs, how much money can OSHA fine an employer for a willful violation?

  a. $250,000
  b. $500,000
  c. $750,000
  d. $1 million

126. When performing safety calculations, especially with regard to potential falls, which of the following correctly represents the gravitational acceleration constant in SI units?

    a. 9.8 meters/second

    b. 9.8 meters/second^2

    c. 32.2 meters/second^2

    d. 32.2 meters/second

127. Which of the following audit-finding classifications is usually considered the most serious?

    a. Conditions adverse to quality

    b. Corrective action issue

    c. Near miss

    d. Tier-1 infraction

128. A safety intervention is defined as a direct action to alter how work is performed with the ultimate goal being to improve worker safety and health. Which of the following would be characterized as a prototypical safety intervention?

    a. DART rate evaluations

    b. Safety incident trend assessments

    c. Design modifications

    d. Submitting a "lessons learned"

129. Per OSHA 29 CFR 1910.21, a "hole" is defined as a gap or open space in a floor, roof, horizontal walking-working surface, or similar surface that is:

    a. At least 12 inches in its least dimension

    b. At least 8 inches in its least dimension

    c. At least 2 inches in its least dimension

    d. At least 1 inch in its least dimension

130. Per ANSI Standards (ANSI/ASSE A1264.2—Slip Resistance on Walking/Working Surfaces), what is a coefficient of friction close to 0.5 typically regarded as?

    a. Extremely slippery

    b. Moderately slippery

    c. Minimally slippery

    d. Not slippery at all

131. ASTM D 120-09 requires that _____ for use in live electrical work exceeding 50 volts must be Type-I.

    a. grounding and bonding materials

    b. rubber-insulating gloves

    c. work boots

    d. hard hats

132. Per OSHA protocol, what must be employed when a construction worker is at least 6 feet above the ground?

    a. Mobile scaffolding platform

    b. Lanyard

    c. Double-rung ladder

    d. Fall-protection equipment

133. An emergency plan should always include procedures for sheltering in place, which need(s) to specifically address which of the following?

a. How to extinguish a small (i.e., manageable) fire during a shelter-in-place event
b. How to evacuate a building during a shelter-in-place event
c. How to shut down all ventilation systems and elevators during a shelter-in-place event
d. How to don appropriate personal protective equipment (PPE) during a shelter-in-place event

134. What is usually considered the proper first step in the conduct of a job safety analysis?

a. To directly observe workers performing their given function or task and to develop an associated list of involved actions
b. To perform a preliminary or cursory evaluation of potential hazards associated with a given function or task
c. To review qualification criteria and records to ensure that worker competency is commensurate with associated responsibilities for a given function or task
d. To review historical event or injury data associated with a given function or task

135. Which of OSHA's programs requires a company to systematically improve its health and safety management system in a well-defined partnership between the employer and workforce?

a. Zero-accident philosophy
b. Integrated safety management
c. Voluntary protection
d. Documented Safety Analysis

136. Structural failures are often due to changes in material compositions or configurations over a period of time. Such changes can ultimately affect a material's strength and/or ductility, thus eventually leading to potential failures. Which of the following conditions or phenomena are often associated with such a scenario?

a. Infrared radiation
b. Electrical conductance
c. Atmospheric inversions
d. Oxidation

137. Injection trauma is a potential hazard associated with the handling of which of the following?

a. Blood-borne pathogens
b. High-pressure fluids
c. syringes
d. Sulfuric acid

138. Which of the following ramp slope angles would be considered marginally acceptable for safely accommodating handicapped access?

a. 15
b. 18
c. 10
d. 12

139. What is the range of the following set of values: 10, 5, 16, 2, 33, 8, 58, 44, and 27?
   a. 17
   b. 56
   c. 22.6
   d. 9

140. An objective measure that is used to assess proactive actions taken to improve organizational performance is typically known as which of the following?
   a. Audit result feedback coefficient
   b. Performance metric
   c. Leading indicator
   d. Lagging indicator

141. Which of the following is considered a vital objective of worker compensation laws?
   a. To put the nation's workforce on an equal legal standing
   b. To prevent workers from filing potentially fraudulent claims
   c. To encourage employers to develop procedures that prevent and reduce accidents
   d. To implement necessary organizational protocols for determining individual culpability due to an incident

142. Which of the following would likely prove to be the best response for a significant near miss that occurs on a worksite?
   a. Immediately issuing a "lessons learned"
   b. Submitting a condition adverse to quality incident report to the organization's safety and health manager
   c. Directing the involved employee(s) to attain a medical check to ensure that no injuries were actually sustained from the near miss
   d. Responding to the near miss with a similar level of rigor and inquiry as that of an actual injury incident by completing a root-cause analysis and developing action plans to prevent potential recurrences

143. Routinely scheduled _____ are a vital component of an effective occupational safety and health program. As such, the frequency of such _____ should be aligned with the degree of risk posed by a subject operation in conjunction with associated regulatory requirements.
   a. NQA-1 audits
   b. Inspections
   c. Industrial hygiene benchmark reviews
   d. ISO-9001 evaluations

144. The statistical expression (standard deviation)² is better known as which of the following?
   a. Chi-squared value
   b. Sigma distribution
   c. Mode
   d. Variance

145. Which of the following is a typical mode of respiratory protection used in the workplace?

    a. Vacuum-fitted respirators
    b. Roughing-filter respirators
    c. Supplied-air respirators
    d. Free-O2 respirators

146. Which of the following should be deemed as a relevant factor when evaluating potential chemical hazards?

    a. Compounds that aren't normally dangerous on their own are normally not dangerous when mixed with other compounds.
    b. Diatomic gases can potentially be more volatile than monatomic gases because they exist at twice the molarity-concentration level of the latter.
    c. Substances that are known hazards may not be considered dangerous at lower concentration levels.
    d. Full-face respiratory protection should always be used when performing assay evaluations to identify chemical constituents.

147. Which of the following is NOT true regarding personal protective equipment (PPE)?

    a. Fit-testing for respirator PPE is a necessity.
    b. PPE is often considered a vital element within the construct of a safety plan.
    c. Nitrile gloves are considered a type of PPE.
    d. PPE should be utilized as a primary means for controlling hazards.

148. Which of the following substances would be most appropriate for extinguishing a fire in energized electrical equipment?

    a. Carbon dioxide
    b. Water
    c. Foam
    d. Copper sulfate

149. Which of the following is considered a repetitive strain injury?

    a. Epicondylitis
    b. Hernia
    c. Colitis
    d. Sciatica

150. Which of the following is a type of ionizing radiation?

    a. Radar waves
    b. Microwaves
    c. Infrared radiation
    d. Beta particles

151. Which of the following actions would likely NOT be considered beneficial to reducing the risk of tripping hazards in the workplace?

    a. Installing ground elevation changes that are no greater than two steps of height differential
    b. Minimizing or eliminating elevation changes between adjoining floor surfaces
    c. Practicing good housekeeping
    d. Using warning signs

152. To effectively follow up on and correct audit findings, subject items should be appropriately organized into which of the following stratified categorizations?

a. Tier I, Tier II, and Tier III
b. Violations, deficiencies, and recommendations
c. Failures, marginalizations, and enhancements
d. Conditions adverse to quality, areas of concern, and improvement opportunities

153. A well-stocked first-aid kit would ordinarily include which of the following?

a. One or more packaged syringes
b. Basic CPR directions
c. Two or more sterile eye dressings
d. Hydrogen peroxide

154. Besides preventing airborne debris from striking workers, what is the other primary function of machine guards?

a. To provide additional machine stability
b. To prevent body parts and clothing from getting caught in pinch points
c. To provide an affixable area for a lockout or tagout process
d. To provide a bonded electrical surface between machine and worker

155. The mathematical product of frequency times consequence is better known as which of the following?

a. Reliability
b. Failure rate
c. Cost
d. Risk

156. Which of the following is true regarding a standard normal data distribution?

a. Exactly 75% of the values fall within ±1 standard deviation of the data set's mean.
b. Exactly 97% of the values fall within ±2 standard deviations of the data set's mean.
c. Exactly 99.7% of the values fall within ±3 standard deviations of the data set's mean.
d. A normal distribution's plot is typically asymmetrically shaped.

157. Which of the following depicts the key difference between a chronic and acute exposure?

a. Acute typically refers to just a singular exposure, whereas chronic is usually marked by several exposures.
b. Health effects suffered from acute exposure cases are almost always considerably more severe than those suffered from chronic exposure cases.
c. Worker compensation payouts are typically much greater for acute cases than chronic cases.
d. An acute exposure is usually somatic in nature, whereas chronic exposures are typically stochastic.

158. An asphyxiant is defined as which of the following?

a. A material that potentially causes bronchial irritation but typically has no long-term hazardous effect on the body

b. A gaseous material that displaces oxygen in air, thus potentially creating a hazardous respiratory environment

c. A substance that can potentially serve as a catalyst for oxygen to support combustion

d. A poisonous gas that affects the nervous system through the eradication of hemoglobin.

159. Which of the following is true with regard to systemic effects to the human body from a hazardous exposure?

a. They are often easily treated.

b. They typically affect the skin and eyes.

c. They usually result in acute death.

d. They usually adversely impact organs and/or biological functions.

160. Which of the following is typically true of burns?

a. A first-degree burn often destroys the skin.

b. A second-degree burn is typically outer-layer superficial with some associated reddening and pain.

c. A third-degree burn usually takes up to a few weeks to heal.

d. A third-degree burn may often exhibit little to no pain.

161. Which are the most common type of workplace injury?

a. Scrapes and cuts

b. Strains and sprains

c. Hairline fractures

d. Contusions

162. What is the most frequently injured part of the body in the workplace?

a. Lower back

b. Ankles

c. Digits (fingers and toes)

d. Head

163. Which of the following is usually a common cause of workplace injuries or incidents?

a. Chemical overexposures

b. Being struck by an object

c. Personal protective equipment (PPE) failure

d. Radiation overexposures

164. Which of the following is true regarding lanyards used within a fall-protection system?

a. Lanyards connect lifelines to pitons.

b. Lanyards connect anchoring points to safety harnesses.

c. Lanyards connect safety belts to fall arrestors.

d. Lanyards connect lifelines to safety belts.

165. On average, approximately 8% of workplace incidents involving lost time are the result of what kind of related injuries?

 a. Workplace violence
 b. Slip or fall
 c. Hand tool
 d. Ergonomic

166. A 1-gallon container of the flammable liquid propylene oxide is found in a storage cabinet at a worksite. Propylene oxide has a flash point of –35°F and a boiling point of 93°F. What flammable liquid class does this chemical fall under?

 a. IB
 b. IIB
 c. IA
 d. IIA

167. A job hazard analysis is performed for an upcoming task in a normal oxygen-rich environment that may likely involve high levels of beryllium and silica dust. Which type of respiratory protection would be deemed MOST appropriate for this planned activity?

 a. An air-purifying, full-face respirator
 b. Supplied air through a hose-mask system or air-line module
 c. An air-supplied suit unit
 d. None provided that worker exposures do not exceed TLVs, TWAs, and STELs

168. A respirator is equipped with a canister that is specifically designed for filtering carbon monoxide gas. Per OSHA guidance, which of the following colors should the canister portray?

 a. Black
 b. Blue
 c. Yellow
 d. Red

169. Which of the following individuals would ideally be the most qualified to measure a variety of radiological hazards in the workplace and resultantly provide recommendations to mitigate such hazards?

 a. Certified health physicist (CHP)
 b. Certified industrial hygienist (CIH)
 c. Certified Safety Professional (CSP)
 d. NSPE-registered nuclear engineer

170. The BCSP requirements for OHST recertification are the reporting of activities every ____ years and a minimum of ____ recertification points.

 a. 2, 15
 b. 3, 40
 c. 5, 20
 d. 7, 35

171. Per OSHA requirements, which of the following would be an acceptable level for illuminating general worksite areas and shops?

a. 2 foot-candles
b. 5 foot-candles
c. 8 foot-candles
d. 12 foot-candles

172. Respirator equipment often undergoes which of the following processes for determining suitability or compatibility with prospective users?

a. Pressure bonding
b. Fit testing
c. Vacuum sealing
d. Intake efficiency

173. Which of the following is a typical hazard associated with welding, cutting, and brazing operations?

a. Acetylene tank explosion
b. Potential eye damage from UV-light
c. Asphyxiation
d. Neuropraxia

174. The Health Insurance Portability and Accountability Act (HIPAA) Privacy Rule covers, by law, which of the following workers' rights?

a. The confidentiality of filing a worker compensation claim
b. The security and privacy of their personal health records
c. That they cannot be terminated due to any incurred health condition
d. To qualify for employer-sponsored health insurance plans regardless of age, sex, or race.

175. What is defined as the average number of lifts performed over a 15-minute period?

a. Lifting median
b. Lifting turnover ratio
c. Lifting index
d. Lifting frequency

176. Which of the following is an example of a compressed-air (pneumatic) tool used at a worksite?

a. Thermocouple
b. Soldering gun
c. Chipper
d. Needle mallet

177. Which of the following is NOT true regarding OSHA inspections?

a. The employer may or may not be advised by the compliance officer of the reason for the inspection.
b. The employer must accompany the compliance officer on the inspection.
c. The compliance officer must show official identification upon an inspection.
d. The compliance officer must assure the employer that any trade secrets observed during the inspection will remain confidential.

178. A company had five recordable injuries with one of them resulting in 40 days of lost time. The total number of hours worked was 216,800. What is the calculated severity rate associated with these statistics?

a. 36.90
b. 0.142
c. 24.08
d. 0.663

179. A weak acid typically has a pH around ___, and a weak base typically has a pH around ___.

a. 0, 7
b. 8, 6
c. 5, 9
d. 1, 14

180. Which of the following agents or substances in the workplace would most likely result in disease or a disorder if repeated exposures occurred?

a. Cadmium
b. Heavy water
c. Glyceryl-oleate
d. Sodium-magnesium silicate

181. Which of the following is an official OSHA violation category?

a. Remedial violation
b. Implicit violation
c. Referral violation
d. Serious violation

182. The term threshold limit value (TLV) in regard to hazardous chemical exposure represents which of the following?

a. An acceptable short-term exposure limit that does not exceed the established time-weighted average for a subject chemical
b. A permissible long-term exposure limit that does not exceed the established time-weighted average for a subject chemical
c. The value at which certain provisions of proposed standards must be initiated, such as periodic employee exposure measurements and training
d. A consensus daily level to which a worker can be exposed over a working lifetime (to a subject chemical) likely without the appearance of adverse health effects

183. A pharmaceutical company is developing a new product to potentially help counteract the effects of lead poisoning. Before it comes to market, however, the company must first seek approval and sanction by which of the following organizations?

a. American Medical Association (AMA)
b. US National Institute of Health (NIH)
c. US Food and Drug Administration (FDA)
d. US Consumer Safety Board (CSB)

184. If an injured worker wishes to file a lawsuit against a company he or she feels is responsible for his or her impaired condition, which of the following attorney types should he or she most likely consult?

a. District attorney
b. Tort infringement
c. Civil
d. State or local attorney-general

185. Which of the following is a typical injury or illness-related metric that is normally tracked by federal agencies?

a. Frequency of nonfatal and nonhospitalized workplace violence incidents
b. Frequency of employee sick days (unrelated to logged incidents)
c. Frequency of medical personnel turnover at a given facility
d. Frequency of restricted duty

186. Which of the following is inclusive of the OSHA Classification System for Occupational Illnesses and Conditions?

a. Impact-related disorders or conditions
b. Radiation-related disorders or conditions
c. Hygiene-related disorders or conditions
d. Psychologically related disorders or conditions

187. Per the US Clean Air Act, which of the following outdoor concentration readings would be considered a violation of National Ambient Air Quality Standards (NAAQS)?

a. 0.5 µg/meter3 of lead (Pb) over a 3-month period
b. 1 ppb of ozone (O_3) over an 8-hour period
c. 0.2 ppm of carbon monoxide (CO) over an 8-hour period
d. 5 ppb of SO2 over a 2-hour period

188. Which of the following US federal agencies is responsible for distributing statistical information pertaining to job-related injuries or illnesses?

a. US National Institute of Health (NIH)
b. US Department of Commerce (DOC)
c. US Bureau of Labor Statistics (BLS)
d. US Bureau of Census (BoC)

189. Which of the following is a typical shape or characterization for a frequency-curve?

a. Elliptical
b. Skewed
c. Figure-eight shaped
d. Hyperbolic

Mometrix

190. A craft employee who was not paying attention while working with a lathe lost the top half of his right index finger in an accident. Corporate Health and Safety management reported the accident to OSHA within 12 hours of the incident. According to OSHA 29 CFR 1904.39, the company is

    a. in compliance with the allowable reporting time frame.
    b. in violation of the allowable reporting time frame.
    c. within the probation zone (i.e., grace period) for the allowable reporting time frame
    d. actually not required to file an OSHA report

191. Which of the following audit-finding classifications is usually considered the LEAST serious?

    a. Condition adverse to quality
    b. Tier-4 marginal infraction
    c. Observation
    d. Opportunity for improvement

192. In the following Cartesian data-point set, which of the following points would be considered an anomaly compared to the others [(−0.4, −1.2), (2, 5.7), (4, 11.8), (7, 20), (9, 28.1), (12, 29), (15, 46.1), and (19, 56)]?

    a. (−0.4, −1.2)
    b. (9, 28.1)
    c. (12, 29)
    d. None

193. Which of the following techniques is NOT typically employed as a tactic for effectively training organization or line management personnel in protocols not specifically laid out in procedural guidance?

    a. Case study deployment
    b. Peer collaboration
    c. Subordinate staging
    d. Role-play

194. Which of the following is a commonly employed conflict resolution strategy used in industry?

    a. Adjudicative resolution
    b. Reciprocal negotiation
    c. Impartial arbitration resolution
    d. Petition resolution

195. Calculations and assessments that evaluate company loss-rate records for establishing _____ rates are conventionally known as experience modifiers.

    a. system failure
    b. worker health insurance
    c. accident or incident
    d. worker compensation

196. What is an office warden typically responsible for during a shelter in place or a building evacuation?

    a. Taking roll call
    b. Contacting emergency officials
    c. Ensuring that all procedures are followed
    d. Activating appropriate alarms

197. According to Frederick Herzberg's theory of behavior, a worker's desired _____ outcomes typically include monetary income, job-security, and safe and comfortable working conditions.

    a. intrinsic
    b. extrinsic
    c. ego-based
    d. survivalist-instinctual

198. A potential workplace-induced hepatitis-C infection from an inadvertent needle-stick event would ultimately be categorized as what on an OSHA 300 form?

    a. Referral case
    b. Tier-I workplace injury case
    c. Infectious disease case
    d. Privacy-case

199. According to Abraham Maslow's hierarchy of needs, which of the following personal facets falls under the need of self-actualization?

    a. Morality
    b. Enhancement of ego
    c. Sense of belonging
    d. Disposition to prejudice

200. Which of the following leadership personalities typically renders decisions on an autonomous basis and closely monitors employees?

    a. Permissive autocrat
    b. Directive democrat
    c. Permissive democrat
    d. Directive autocrat

Answer Key and Explanations

1. D: Effective worksite safety inspections are usually conducted by inspectors who are independent entities that do not have a direct affiliation with the organization or entity being inspected and are likewise typically conducted by personnel who have expert-level knowledge, training, and/or experience within the subject area(s) being inspected. Furthermore, inspections can either be unscheduled or scheduled, but unscheduled inspections typically provide better insights than scheduled ones.

2. C: A robust incident reporting system (IRS) typically includes reporting mechanisms for properly differentiating and distinguishing between and among incident severity categories. Processes for commencing worker compensation claims and submitting "lessons learned" are typically independent of IRS functions. Remote electronic access capabilities in the field, although a desirable option if available, are not a mandatory element of such a system and are thus typically seldom implemented.

3. A: A major benefit that usually results from undergoing an external audit is the attainment of benchmarking information (per audit findings) against that of industry competitors who have undergone similar audits.

4. A: Frostbite is a dangerous condition that can occur as a result of prolonged exposure to extreme cold. It manifests when the temperature of body tissues falls below the freezing point of those tissues (essentially below the freezing point of water). In such instances, tissue damage usually occurs and can potentially lead to the loss of damaged toes or fingers in severe cases (digital frostbite). In addition, the victim may or may not feel pain associated with the onset of such a condition and likewise may also encounter skin that turns gray or white in color. In contrast, chilblains are another type of health hazard that can occur from overexposure to cold; however, these usually result from a combined exposure to cold and humidity and are typically depicted by toe redness, inflammation, itching, and occasional blistering.

5. B: Light metals such as aluminum, lithium, and beryllium are typically not employed as effective shielding materials for protection against exposure to gamma or X-ray radiation. The best shielding materials against these types of ionizing radiations include lead, concrete, uranium, and water.

6. C: Workplace hazards may arise in a number of different ways during the conduct of maintenance activities, including not adhering to consistent maintenance schedules; utilizing incorrect or outdated maintenance schedules; using poorly written maintenance procedures that do not clearly convey necessary step-by-step protocols; and executing work functions on systems that are not of a user-friendly design for maintenance (e.g., limited access or service locations).

7. A: The tangent of angle $\angle ABC$ is by definition equal to b/a, which is the opposite side over the adjacent side.

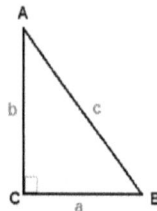

8. C: Several methods can be deployed in the workplace for significantly reducing hazardous noise levels; such strategies can include the use of double-barrier hearing personal protective equipment (PPE), whereby both earplugs and earmuffs are worn by workers, and installation of sound-absorbent materials, decreasing vibrational frequencies and sound flow rates and redirecting sound sources away from workers. Attempting to integrate white-noise (background) sources within a noisy work environment can actually add to gross ambient noise levels and is thus not recommended.

9. C: Gloves made from leather or cowhide material are conventionally used for effective protection against welding sparks. Gloves made from other (synthetic) materials (e.g., neoprene or rubber) are widely used for protection against chemical agents.

10. C: The number 21 is the statistical median of the data set: 6, 13, 15, 15, 18, 24, 28, 33, 51, and 66. If there is an even number of values in a data set (such as 10 for this case), the median is the average of the two middle values of the set. Thus, (18+24)/2 = 21. If there were an odd number of values, the median would be the value that has the same number of values that are both above and below it. For instance, if the data set instead consisted of the following nine values—6, 13, 15, 15, 18, 24, 33, 51 and 66—the median would be 18 because it has four values that are greater and four values that are lesser.

11. B: Determining how much monetary value to place on a human life is usually regarded as the most difficult challenge associated with the rendering of a cost-benefit analysis. Other facets such as the performance of associated risk assessments, determining long-term cost savings of proposed safety enhancements, and formulating or defending design-basis criteria, however, can also exhibit a certain degree of inherent difficulty.

12. A: A GANTT chart is often utilized within the realm of project management to effectively illustrate a project schedule. It typically depicts how much time should be spent on each project step and prioritizes the order in which those steps should be completed as well as key milestones, available float, and the project's critical path.

13. C: In regard to the concept of continual improvement, performance improvement should be sought at a variety of paces, depending on the circumstances at hand. A reasonable amount of time should always be allocated for a performance improvement process to take hold and should not be approached with a large-scale, quick-fix mentality. In addition, it is value-added to effectively integrate "lessons-learned" programs with continual improvement programs to the highest extent practicable.

14. B: The plan-do-check-act model is highly utilized within industrial occupational safety and health regimes and work-control programs to ensure that work is appropriately planned and safely performed.

15. A: The purpose of an accident investigation is to prevent future accidents and return the company to confident functioning. The sooner an accident's root cause(s) is/are discovered, the sooner these lessons can be shared with the subject organization for preventing recurrences. A prompt response to an accident also sends a message of robust corporate response and engagement, and witness accounts are usually more reliable earlier as opposed to later.

16. A: Typically implemented protocols for protecting workers from blood-borne pathogens include requiring hand-washing after removal of glove personal protective equipment (PPE); training workers to assume that all bodily fluids are potentially infectious; and not permitting eating or drinking in areas where pathogens may be present. Regular employee health screenings and medical monitoring do(es) not, per se, protect workers from blood-borne pathogens, although they may be able to identify potentially infectious diseases that employees may be (unaware) carriers of. Requiring infectious personnel to wear additional PPE as compared to other employees or requesting that infectious personnel disclose certain health conditions may be in violation of HIPAA requirements.

17. C: Heinrich's 10 Axioms of Workplace Safety include the following: Most accidents are usually correlated to unsafe worker behavior; knowing why people work unsafely can usually assist in producing appropriate corrective measures; and management usually plays a vital role within the realm of accident prevention. Additional axioms include these: Unsafe worker actions do not always quickly result in an incident; safety should be the ultimate responsibility of management; and most accidents are, in fact, preventable.

18. D: According to the Errors in Management Systems theory (developed by Juran and Deming), approximately 85% of errors in the workplace are usually the result of insufficient management procedures and/or processes.

19. A: If a work area has dimensions of 30 ft x 18 ft x 8 ft, the shortest amount of time it could potentially take for the entire supply of air in the room to (hypothetically) be completely exchanged via an air-exchanger HVAC system that operates at a rate of 60 cfm would be approximately 1.2 hours. This is calculated via the following:

Total air exchange time = $4320 \text{ ft}^3 \times \frac{1 \text{ min}}{60 \text{ ft}^3} = 72 \text{ min} = 1.2 \text{ hours}$

20. B: Types of hearing hazards associated with exposure(s) to loud noise include shifts in threshold due to short- or long-term noise exposure; acoustical traumas caused by a sudden, extreme loud noise; and tinnitus (ringing in the ears) caused by short- or long-term noise exposure.

21. C: Nip-point hazards (in which body parts or clothing can become ensnared) are inherently associated with the functionality of many machine components, especially those that rotate toward one another or toward a stationary component. Examples of nip-prone items include gears, pulleys, rollers, belts, and bearings. Bushings have no ensnaring capability; actuators are essentially fully enclosed (encased) motor mechanisms; and guards are structures installed for protecting against an ensnarement-type incident.

22. C: There are four fundamental established tenets of ergonomics across general industry: whenever possible, the job should be changed and not the worker; people differ from one another; people should work smart; and people are more appropriate for some tasks than machines are and vice versa.

23. D: Utilizing wires that are not excessively long is considered a robust physical control against electrical hazards. The longer a wire is, the more electrical resistance tends to build within, and thus a higher level of associated heat (and potential for fire) is produced. Other physical controls against electrical hazards include using insulation, conduits, and barriers to provide a buffer between electrical sources and personnel; ensuring proper connections of conductors; and properly locating and situating high-voltage equipment.

24. C: Fully assessing confined-space hazards prior to entry is proper protocol, as opposed to only assessing them after entry and work have commenced. Moreover, use of a buddy system is an excellent control strategy to employ for protecting against hazards associated with confined-space work as well as sufficient worker training; installation of accessible fire-suppression equipment; and ensuring that sufficient ventilation is available within the space.

25. B: Chemical irritants are compounds that can adversely (and temporarily) affect the skin (dermatitis) and mucus membranes as well as the eyes and respiratory tract. They do not typically cause permanent tissue damage as a result of normal exposure(s). Examples of irritants include the likes of chlorine, ammonia, nitrogen dioxide, and ozone.

26. A: Workplace biohazards can be either animal- or plant-based; can be either toxic or allergenic-based in nature; can include certain types of bacteria, viruses, or fungi; and are usually transmitted by some type of direct contact with bodily or plant-based fluids.

27. D: TRIR measures all types of OSHA recordable incidents while the other options deal with subsets of recordable incidents.

28. A: There are several preventative and remedial measures that can be implemented in the workplace to normally combat sick-office syndrome. Chief examples include maintaining low building humidity levels; regularly cleaning furniture, carpets, and floors; regularly discarding accumulated condensation from HVAC collection systems; and regularly changing out HVAC system air filters. The invocation of extreme measures such as employee isolation, furniture replacement, or floor-material change outs would typically be implemented only for localized extreme cases of epidemic-type proportions.

29. D: There are four regularly utilized principles typically exercised in workplaces for the deployment of proper workstation configurations; these include usage sequence, usage frequency, usage functionality, and usage importance.

30. D: Building evacuation plans should be designed so that personnel still know where to exit in virtual total darkness; they should likewise include use and guidance of alarm systems as a mode of communication and should also specify locations of outdoor mustering areas. In contrast, emergency plans and protocols typically address items related to emergency response team activations, sheltering in place, and fire response procedures.

31. C: Although OSHA does not administer specific indoor air quality (IAQ) standards, it does maintain a cadre of general ventilation protocols as well as guidance regarding specific air contaminants that can potentially spawn IAQ issues. As such, recirculated-air system operational requirements must include, at a minimum, the following: Recirculated air must undergo regular sampling and evaluation to verify that cleaning systems are functioning normally; contaminated air must be routed outdoors in the event of an incident; air-cleaning systems must have audial and visual warning indicators to advise personnel of potential issues (no specified illumination or loudness requirements); and secondary filtration modules must maintain an efficiency at least equal to that of a subject system's primary filtration modules (there are no requirements for potential tertiary modules).

32. B: Types of electrical-switching devices that are typically used in the workplace for preventing access to hazardous electrical areas, or for altogether interrupting electrical power, include interlocks, cutouts, and lockouts. Interlocks essentially prevent employee access to energized equipment or work areas; cutouts automatically trip power to electrical equipment when a certain temperature is reached; and lockouts prevent equipment from being switched into the on mode.

33. C: On average, about 25% of worker compensation claims are typically associated with lower-back injuries, with most of these being attributed to poor lifting techniques or lifting too much weight.

34. A: Normlessness-powerlessness-mindlessness is an archetypal set of worker behavioral dynamics that often result from increased levels of industrial automation (and potential associated workforce reductions) within a workplace setting. All of these behaviors can ultimately lead to lessened quality and productivity as well as a higher incidence of workplace accidents.

35. D: There are three general approaches used in industry for asbestos abatement: encapsulation, enclosure, and removal. Encapsulation involves spraying asbestos with a binding-type sealant that will keep the subject material in place (i.e., virtually eliminating the potential of it becoming airborne); enclosure involves emplacing permanent air-tight walls around the asbestos material; and removal ultimately entails a four-step process of temporary isolation, negative pressure, application of an immobilization solution, and disposal.

36. A: Ventilation systems are designed to provide a number of benefits to indoor working environments; namely, they help reduce the buildup of carbon dioxide, they help reduce dust levels, they maintain air temperatures at comfortable levels, they reduce unpleasant ambient odors, and they help maintain flammable vapor concentrations and contaminant levels below hazardous thresholds.

37. B: The first step that should be implemented in the construct of a robust facility emergency plan should be the assemblage of a plan team from a variety of organizational functions and disciplines. This scenario inevitably supplies a diverse set of viewpoints and areas of expertise that will ultimately result in the development of a stronger overall plan. The crafting of subject documentation such as a plan mission statement and a draft disaster-response procedure should commence after the plan team has been assembled.

38. A: The most imperative reason for conducting a workplace safety analysis is typically to help avoid accidents by determining what hazards exist and what controls are required to avoid them. In addition, formal safety analyses (e.g., safety analysis reports [SARs] and technical safety requirements [TSRs]) are often mandated by law or by contractual agreement. Moreover, workplace safety analyses can in the long-term result in potentially lower worker compensation premiums (due to lower incident frequencies) as well as assisting with voluntary protection program (VPP) certifications.

39. C: The Five-Why method is universally regarded as an extremely effective method or model for conducting a root-cause analysis. This approach essentially advocates the use of five consecutive, logically connected, why questions that are used to ultimately reach the root cause or justification behind an incident.

40. C: Electrical insulators are materials that inhibit the free flow of electricity. Good insulating materials include oil, rubber, wood, plastics, and glass. Materials that are not good electrical insulators (i.e., conductors) include iron, copper, aluminum, precious metals, and salt water.

41. B: Electrical fires often occur due to electrical short outs (i.e., shorts) or poor connections. Furthermore, such fires are also often initiated due to an overflow of current through a material. The resulting excess heat that is generated in such overflow scenarios can ultimately ignite nearby flammable items.

42. C: The overall calculated annual risk of an accident event that has a frequency of 0.0005/year and an associated consequence of 1.4 fatalities is derived by multiplying the two values together. Risk is equal to the product of frequency times consequence. Thus, (0.0005/year) x (1.4 fatalities) = 0.00070 fatalities/year.

43. D: A histogram most closely resembles a bar graph in appearance and structure. Each vertically oriented bar of a histogram typically depicts a specific data set that falls under the requirements of that particular bar's regime. The larger the number of data points included within a subject bar, the taller the bar appears.

44. D: A worst-case project choice from a cost-benefit standpoint is one that has the lowest possible monetary ratio of benefits to costs; such a case would entail a cumulative net benefit amount of $0, which would therefore result in an associated ratio equal to zero.

45. D: Statistical correlation coefficients entail several distinct characteristics, including the following: They represent how strong of a functional relationship exists between a linear regression equation's two variables; coefficients of +1 reflect a positive correlation between variables; coefficients of –1 reflect a negative correlation between variables; and the determination of such values can provide a robust indicator as to whether a given equation depicting a best-fit line is appropriately accurate. In contrast, a coefficient equal to zero reflects a total absence of correlation between variables.

46. C: There are three primary categories normally evaluated within the realm of accident prevention; these include accident financial impacts (i.e., monetary risks), accident severities or consequences, and accident probabilities.

47. B: If the ground supports an object with 12.5 Newtons, the object weighs 12.5 Newtons. The mass of the object can be calculated from the weight (force) using the fundamental mechanics equation F = ma, whereby F = force, m = mass, and a = acceleration (in this particular case, an acceleration due to gravity [9.8 m/s^2]). In terms of the subject SI units, 1N = (1kg)(1m/s^2). Thus, the mass = Force/acceleration. 12.5 N/9.8 m/s^2 = 1.28 kilograms.

48. C: A type-A-rated fire extinguisher is effective against a fire that is trash, wood, or paper based (i.e., ordinary solid combustibles). Nonconductive extinguishing agents such as monoammonium phosphate and film-forming foam are typically used to fight this type of fire because of their smothering or blanketing and nonconductive natures. They are also effective at suppressing fire-induced vapors.

49. A: Anti-C/respirator tandems are most effective at protecting workers from all potential alpha exposure pathways as well as from most low-energy beta sources. They are not, however, effective at attenuating external gamma radiation (or neutron radiation); however, they are effective at preventing internal uptakes of such emanating sources. The primary function of Anti-C personal protective equipment (PPE) is to prevent worker contamination, whereas respirators are specifically employed to protect workers from uptakes via inhalation and/or ingestion.

50. D: In EPA-space, TSCA stands for the Toxic Substances Control Act. This act, first promulgated in 1976, is the primary US federal law that assesses and regulates new commercial chemicals before they enter into the marketplace; regulates the handling of presently existent chemicals that may pose an unreasonable risk to public health or to the environment; and regulates the overall distribution and use of potentially dangerous chemicals.

51. C: 1 M (molar) nitric acid (HNO_3), 2 M hydrochloric acid (HCl), and 4 M hydrofluoric acid (HF) are appreciably more caustic and thus pose a much greater hazard to human health than 4 M acetic acid ($C_2H_4O_2$). The former three acids are defined as "strong acids; the latter acid (acetic), however, although having a molar concentration that is higher than that for HNO_3 and HCl in this instance, is a very weak acid.

52. D: The fire tetrahedron consists of four essential elements: oxygen, fuel, heat, and the resulting perpetual, exothermic-based chain-reaction. The chain reaction maintaining the fire will continue until at least one of the first three elements (oxygen, fuel, or heat) is eliminated. Smoke is not an element of the fire tetrahedron but is of course a most dangerous (and often fatal) by-product resulting from a fire event.

53. A: There are several established parametric acronyms implemented and exercised by US regulatory and guidance agencies in regard to chemical hazard exposure limits. The most notable include the following: short-term exposure limits (STELs) and threshold limit values (TLVs) set forth by the American Conference of Governmental Industrial Hygienists (ACGIH) and the Occupational Safety and Health Administration (OSHA). In addition, permissible exposure limits (PELs) are set forth by OSHA, and recommended exposure limits (RELs) are set forth by the National Institute of Occupational Safety and Health (NIOSH).

54. A: The Occupational Safety and Health (OSH) Act of 1970 (and amendments) requires that employers provide safety and health training to their (new and existing) employees. The OSH Act is administered and enforced by OSHA.

55. B: The US Department of Transportation (USDOT) should be immediately notified (first) in the event of any accidental release of hazardous materials during transportation. This includes, but is not limited to, any chemical, radiological, or biohazardous media.

56. D: For the six variables conventionally applied (H-V-D-F-A-C) in determining recommended weight limits, D stands for vertical travel distance of a lift. The other variables are denoted by the following: H = load horizontal distance; V = vertical location; F = lift frequency; A = load angle; and C = hand-to-load coupling.

57. B: Natural-occurring hazards that can probabilistically lead to fires and/or explosions within or around workplace locations include floods, hurricanes, earthquakes, tornadoes, lightning, and droughts.

58. A: Inhalation is by far the most hazardous pathway for potential radon intake or uptake. Radon's high-energy alpha particle tracks easily damage thin lung (epithelial) tissues much more readily and severely than any other body organ. Radon is universally accepted as the number-two source of lung cancer behind cigarette smoke.

59. C: State regulatory permits are normally required for storm water (runoff), facility air emissions, wastewater, radioactive materials, hazardous waste (management), and onsite petroleum storage.

60. B: When a chemical reaction arises from an acid and a base being mixed together, water and salt are conventionally yielded as the reaction products. For example, when hydrofluoric acid and potassium hydroxide are combined, the result is water and potassium fluoride.

61. C: A fitness-for-duty assessment, often required by employers, is used to evaluate whether a candidate or present employee is (or is not) able to perform required job functions due to physical or psychological limitations. Such evaluations are often reassessed on a periodic basis through the use of medical monitoring programs or similar mechanisms.

62. C: Death via smoke inhalation usually accounts for the highest proportion of fire-related fatalities. This is usually due to two primary contributory factors: (1) toxic fumes in the smoke can render victims unconscious (and hence, immobile) in a matter of seconds, and (2) because a fire consumes considerable oxygen within an event area, there is resultantly less oxygen available for respiration, which promotes an even greater likelihood a victim will lose consciousness even more quickly in such an environment.

63. D: Several adverse physical conditions can manifest over time from excessive exposure(s) to vibrating machinery; namely, white-finger syndrome, diminished hand dexterity or grip, carpal tunnel syndrome, or possibly even permanent loss of sensation in the extremities or digits due to nerve damage.

64. B: An endeavor to uncover and reduce hazards that may be at hand for product or system users, as well as to those who are accountable for their maintenance, is conventionally known as an Occupational Health Hazard Assessment. Such assessments also usually attempt to evaluate ways to reduce risks or impacts resulting from such hazards if an associated undesirable event was to subsequently unfold.

65. A: A Hazard and Operability Study (HAZOP) is a structured evaluation of a planned or existing endeavor or process in an attempt to identify and analyze potential issues that may ultimately manifest in risks to workers, equipment, and/or operational efficiencies.

66. B: There are several key components to proper seating posture within workstation environments, which include maintaining the forearms in a parallel configuration to the floor, keeping one's chin in a downward-type position, and keeping both feet flat on the floor. In addition, footrests may be used as appropriate, however, to facilitate proper posture and worker comfort. Moreover, appropriate computer screen distances in the range of 16 to 28 inches should regularly be employed dependent upon the user's individual ophthalmological needs.

67. D: Numerous materials and agents are utilized as fire suppressants dependent on the type of extinguishing device used and, thus, the type of fire at hand. Such materials include potassium bicarbonate, monoammonium phosphate, carbon dioxide, sodium bicarbonate, potassium chloride, halon, and of course, water.

68. D: Within the realm of statics and mechanics, a structure is considered statically indeterminate if the number of forces (variables) exceeds the number of available equilibrium equations. In this working example, there are four separate forces placed upon the static hoist, and yet there are only three independent equilibrium equations depicting the relationships of these forces; the object's condition is hence considered to be statically indeterminate because the equations cannot be solved to render a single definitive value attributable to each force variable.

69. B: General ergonomic requirements, per OSHA, are enforced per the Administration's General Duty Clause, Section 5(a)(1).

70. C: There are presently five separate categories or classes of fire extinguisher technologies available in modern-day industry that are designed to handle different types of fires. The five alpha-based codes that denote these classes are A, B, C, D, and K. Class A (green-triangle symbol) is for typical combustibles such as paper, wood, and plastic; Class B (red-square symbol) is for combustible liquids such as oil, grease, or gasoline; Class C (blue-circle symbol) is for live electrical

191

equipment or highly conductive materials; Class D (yellow-decagon symbol) is for combustible metals such as sodium, potassium, and magnesium; and Class K (black-hexagon symbol) is for cooking oils and fats (hence, the K class stands for kitchen).

71. D: Per EPA guidelines, a robust environmental management system (EMS) can entail several distinct elements, including maintaining in-house environmental databases, maintaining employee environmental-related competencies, regularly evaluating potential environmental impacts associated with the EMS, regularly assessing associated EMS legal requirements, and regularly reviewing an organization's environmental objectives.

72. B: The fellow-servant rule is an often-utilized defense posture corporate entities implement against on-the-job injury claims filed by employees. Dependent upon the situation and extent of litigation, however, other legal defense approaches such as contributory negligence and assumption of risk may also potentially be utilized by employers who endeavor to protect their corporate interests against such claims.

73. B: The National Environmental Policy Act (NEPA) of 1969 typically renders documentation that assesses potential environmental impacts resulting from major proposed actions at federal, state, and local levels. Such documents and determinations usually include Environmental Impact Statements (EISs), environmental assessments (EAs), findings of no significant impact (FONSIs), and categorical exclusions (CXs). In contrast, Documented Safety Analyses are typically facility safety-basis-related assessments that are mandated by government agencies (such as the US Nuclear Regulatory Commission and the US Department of Energy) for a subject facility to be licensed for operation.

74. A: If a storage shelf has a weight-limit capacity of 200 pounds and a safe utilization surface-area of 30 feet^2, it will be able to handle no more than three 27 feet^3 square-shaped 25-pound boxes, with no stacking of boxes being permitted. This is determined via the fact that any of a square-shaped box's six sides will have a surface area of 9 feet^2 (3 feet x 3 feet), thus, only three boxes can fit (equaling a total surface area of 27 feet^2) within the 30 feet^2 shelf area. In addition, the three boxes together weigh only 75 pounds, which is less than the prescribed 200-pound total limit.

75. C: Per industry standards, the minimum required net efficiency for a filtration system to be categorized as high-efficiency particulate arrestance (HEPA) is typically 99.97%, with greater than 3 μm diameter (AMAD) particles.

76. C: The International Organization for Standardization (ISO) 9000 Standard is the most widely utilized guidance system in the United States for employing robust quality management and assurance programs.

77. C: Within the realms of environmental management and the US Clean Air Act, the term RACT conventionally stands for reasonably available control technology.

78. B: A noise dosimeter is a commonly used device for measuring potentially hazardous noise levels in industrial settings. It is usually employed in a manner that continuously processes noise levels throughout the duration of a work shift (in a particular work area) and then provides an equivalent cumulative quantity at the end of that shift, depicting what a worker's total noise exposure would be in that area.

79. A: A disaster recovery plan should designate a recovery coordinator who ultimately determines what recovery actions need to be taken and furthermore assigns responsibilities for achieving such actions.

80. D: There are several key aspects or factors that are normally considered when designing an optimal ergonomic environment for older and aging workers; these typically include providing state-of-the-art ergonomic seating and chairs to accommodate posture changes or deterioration; enhancing lighting or illumination levels in work areas for improved visibility; and providing hand tools that include power grips to compensate for decreased strength and dexterity.

81. D: The primary EPA legislative mechanism that enforces overall standards for potable water quality is the Safe Drinking Water Act.

82. D: The US FDA is responsible for protecting the public at large from potential hazards associated with the use of all pharmaceutical products as well as sold foodstuffs, organics, cosmetics, or any other products available for curative applications.

83. A: Typical parameters shown or used on a crane load chart for calculating safe load limits include a crane's boom angle, a crane's boom length, and a crane's operating radius.

84. D: The four colors of the NFPA 704 Diamond System are yellow (right side of the diamond, depicting instability level), blue (left side of the diamond, depicting health hazard level), red (top side of the diamond, depicting fire hazard level), and white (bottom side of the diamond, depicting special hazard levels for oxidizers and water reactions). Numbers from 0 to 4 are provided in each segment depicting the level of hazard (0 = lowest and 4 = highest).

85. D: The OSHA Classification System for Occupational Illnesses and Conditions includes several categorical facets, including respiratory- and lung-related disorders or conditions, radiation-related disorders or conditions, skin-related disorders or conditions, toxic-related disorders or conditions, and repetitive-motion or ergonomic-related disorders or conditions.

86. C: The US Bureau of Labor Statistics is ultimately charged with and responsible for distributing statistical information pertaining to job-related injuries or illnesses. Other agencies, however, such as the US Occupational Safety and Health Administration and the US National Institute of Occupational Safety and Health often cite or reference such published statistics in support of their missions, campaigns, outreach, and enforcement initiatives.

87. B: Per the US Nuclear Regulatory Commission's mandated annual worker dose limit of 5 rem (re: 10 CFR 20), 10% of this limit would be received by a worker over a calendar year if he or she was exposed to an average daily 2 millirem dose (for an 8-hour workday) over a 2,000 hour work year. This is derived via: (2 millirem/8 hours)(2,000 hour)(1 rem/1000 millirem) = 0.5 rem, which is 10% of 5 rem.

88. D: The longest sequence of activities in a project plan that all must be completed on time for a given project, as a whole, to be completed on time is known as the project's critical path.

89. D: The scope of a job safety analysis (JSA) typically entails several facets, including the overall integration of safety principles with job practices associated with a given task; the identification of potential hazards associated with a given task; and the notation of safety recommendations associated with a given task.

90. B: Hand tools should always be designed such that the handle's center of gravity is properly aligned with the center of the hand when held. In addition, the conventionally recommended upper weight limit for industrial hand tools is 1.0 kilogram (2.2 pounds, with potentially lighter tools (with power grips) ultimately recommended for older workers.

91. C: Dimethyl ether is a Class-IA (highest flammability class) flammable liquid and is thus considerably more flammable than nitromethane, paraffin oil (kerosene), and biodiesel, which are Class-IC or lower flammables. The flammable liquid classification system (i.e., Classes I-III) is used extensively by the US NFPA, US EPA, US DOT, and OSHA.

92. D: Faulty electrical systems and connections (e.g., poorly connected or worn wiring, overloaded circuits, and inadequate heat dispensation) are usually responsible for causing the preponderance of workplace fires. Other noteworthy fire initiators include worker error, flammable or combustible material misuse or improper storage, general negligence, and arson.

93. D: The fossil-fuel (oil, gas, coal, etc.) industry is regularly associated with the highest frequency of workplace fire- and explosion-related deaths in the United States. This of course is directly correlated with the highly volatile characteristics of the petroleum-based materials that are handled. Other industries that likewise handle (or use) high quantities of volatile materiel (such as chemical-processing, mining or explosive ordnance fabrication) also have a higher-than-average frequency of fire- and explosion-related incidents.

94. B: Hydrogen has three separate nuclides (isotopes) that exist in nature: protium (one proton and two neutrons), deuterium (one proton and one neutron), and tritium (one proton and two neutrons), with only the latter (tritium) being radioactive. Tritium has approximately a 12-year half-life and undergoes its disintegration via beta decay.

95. C: A back belt is a device used in the workplace for reducing the forces on the spine during lifting tasks via increased abdominal pressure and the stimulation of associated core muscles as well as by stiffening and immobilizing the spine itself.

96. B: There are numerous recommended strategies per the National Institute of Occupational Safety and Health (NIOSH) for implementing an effective ergonomics program. Such strategies include regularly identifying and implementing ergonomic controls in the workplace, acquiring and analyzing ergonomic-related data (e.g., MSD injury and incident data reviews), and offering a formidable ergonomics training program. As for potential intervention strategies, these should be conducted prior to the onset of a condition and a resulting diagnosis.

97. B: Carpal-tunnel syndrome is an unpleasant and often distressing condition that affects the hands and fingers, caused by the compression of a major nerve that passes over the carpal bones through a passage (tunnel) in the wrist. Several symptoms that normally indicate the presence of carpal-tunnel syndrome include numbness and tingling in the thumb, index, middle, and/or ring fingers; wrist pain; wrist stiffness; and weakened grip. The pinky finger, however, is usually not affected given that it is not connected to the subject condition's neural pathway.

98. B: There are usually three separate classification levels typically utilized for categorizing deficiencies noted during internal or external audits (or assessments). These are (in order of severity): conditions adverse to quality (nonconformances), corrective actions (areas for concern), and opportunities for improvement (observations). In addition, noteworthy practices can also be highlighted as a "yardstick" or guide for helping implement potential improvements in designated areas.

99. A: The recommended upper weight or force limit of an object that is to be horizontally pushed or pulled from a seated position is a 29-pound force.

100. D: Several parameters are normally evaluated when characterizing soil quality; these include the soil's conductivity, porosity, moisture content, solubility or saturation levels, mineral levels, acidity or alkalinity (i.e., pH), and potential contaminant levels.

101. A: There are several technologies employed in industry that effectively eliminate biologically based water contaminants such as bacteria. These namely include ultraviolet light, chlorination, and ozone.

102. C: The end result of a potential electrocution incident is generally determined by the following: the duration of time to which a person is exposed to a subject current, the quantity of current that passes through the body, and the actual path through the body that the current proceeds.

103. C: Per OSHA 29 CFR 1910.95, a noise hazard control program must be set into effect for workers who are regularly exposed to an 8-hour time-weighted average of 85 dB or greater.

104. C: Per OSHA 29 CFR 1910.1001, an employer shall ensure that no worker is exposed to an airborne asbestos concentration exceeding of 0.1 fiber per centimeter^3 of air over an 8-hour time-weighted average period.

105. B: Certain attributes for hazardous waste are stipulated and codified within EPA regulations (40 CFR 261, Subpart C) for special designation. The four properties, in order, are ignitability (# D001), corrosivity (#D002), reactivity (#D003), and toxicity (#s D004-D043). Mutagenicity, teratogenicity, and volatility are not designated as codified characteristics per 40 CFR 261, Subpart C.

106. B: Lifting index (LI) measures the physical stress associated with the lifting of an object. As LI increases, the chance of a resulting injury also increases. LI is calculated by dividing the load weight by the recommended weight limit (RWL).

107. B: A body harness consists of straps attached to other components of a personal fall system. In case of a fall incident, the subject straps mainly distribute the fall-arrest forces over the chest, shoulders, waist, thighs, and pelvis. A properly designed (and donned) harness should yield minimal impacts to the lower back, arms, and feet.

108. A: Recommended Weight Limit (RWL) is the weight that healthy workers can lift for up to 8 hours without causing musculoskeletal injuries. It is calculated as the mathematical product of load constant, horizontal multiplier, vertical multiplier, distance multiplier, asymmetric multiplier, frequency multiplier, and coupling multiplier.

109. D: The incident-injury ratio Heinrich developed is 300:29:1 (none:minor:major). Extrapolating out to 1,000 potential incidents, this equates to proportional ratios of 909:88:3. The ratio relationship essentially exemplifies the notion (from a statistical basis) that an attentive manager or foreman usually has numerous opportunities to improve a safety program or regimen before a serious accident potentially occurs.

110. B: Total case incident rate (TCIR) is a health and safety measure that represents the total number of OSHA recordable injury cases in a year and is altogether weighted by the number of total hours worked by subject employees during that year. The measure is primarily used for comparison (or benchmarking) between entities in similar industries.

111. B: Falls at construction worksites usually represent the highest source of fatalities (about one-third). Other major fatality sources at construction worksites include those from transportation-related incidents (about 25%), contact with objects and equipment (about 20%), and exposure to harmful substances (about 15%).

112. D: Although any amount of electrical current over 10 milliamperes typically produces painful to severe shock, death usually does not occur at levels below 75 milliamperes. A current exposure of 0.2 amperes (i.e., 200 milliamperes) nearly always results in a fatality.

113. C: The ring test evaluates sound emanating from a grinding wheel. The test is conducted via lightly tapping the wheel with a nonmetallic material. An undamaged wheel emits a clear ringing tone, while a damaged wheel will not. The ring test should not, however, be conducted on wheels that have a diameter of 10 centimeters or less, plugs and cones, mounted wheels, segment wheels, or inserted nut and projecting stud-disc wheels.

114. B: Although all involved entities within an organization should take ownership and accountability for all facets of job site safety, it is ultimately the employer's responsibility to ensure that only well-maintained and operable hand and power tools are utilized at a job site.

115. B: Under current US laws for worker compensation, there are four potential injury categories: (1) partial—when an employee can still work but is unable to perform all duties of a job due to an incurred injury; (2) total—when an employee is fully unable to work or perform substantial duties on the job; (3) temporary—when an employee is expected to fully recover from an incurred injury; and (4) permanent—when an employee will suffer effects from an injury for the rest of his or her life.

116. B: Heat stroke occurs when the body's temperature regulation system fails and sweating becomes inadequate or altogether stops entirely. It is an emergency medical condition and if immediate treatment is not administered, brain damage or death is very likely to occur. Signs and symptoms of heat stroke may include face redness, euphoria, confusion, restlessness, irritability, chills or shivering, disorientation, cessation of sweating, very hot skin, erratic behavior, collapse, unconsciousness, convulsions, and a core body temperature that exceeds 104°F. To prevent the occurrence of heat stroke, workers should steadily adapt themselves to their high-temperature work environments, follow an appropriate work-rest cycle, drink and maintain adequate fluids, and follow a proper diet.

117. C: The ISO 14001 environmental management system is built on upon the plan-do-check-act model. The language of the system advises that a working organization (1) establish an environmental policy; (2) thoroughly commit to compliance with all applicable environmental regulations; (3) satisfactorily communicate their environmental program policies to their employees; and (4) periodically conduct audits to assess program compliance levels.

118. D: The only stated condition that would be characteristic of a hazardous atmospheric environment is the presence of a flammable gas at a concentration of 50 percent of its lower flammability limit (LFL). Acceptable or normal atmospheric concentrations of carbon dioxide are typically less than 600 parts per million, and atmospheric oxygen concentrations are considered normal between a range of 19.5 and 23.5 percent in air.

119. A: Per OSHA 29 CFR 1904.33, the time requirement for retention of documents (e.g., OSHA Form 301) is designated to be 5 years following the end of the calendar year that the records cover.

120. A: The OHSAS 18000 series of occupational health and safety management system guidance sets a protocol basis for successfully controlling the overall health and safety of workers. The purpose of such a system is to implement a systemic approach that is commensurate to the manner in which an organization manages its health and safety programs, with the overall goal being to proactively identify and respond to potential risks before an event occurs.

121. B: Per OSHA 29 CFR 1910.211(b), cut-off wheels are recommended only for use on fully guarded and specially designed machines. A wheel with a diameter of 9 inches (i.e., within the range of 6 to 12 inches) can cut a material with a maximum thickness of ¼ inch.

122. A: Per OSHA 29 CFR 1910.1025, the permissible exposure limit (PEL) for lead is 50 micrograms per cubic meter (50 ug/meter^3) of air, averaged over 8 hours. This means that the employer shall ensure that no employee is exposed to lead concentrations greater than 50 micrograms per cubic meter of air over an 8-hour average period. Action levels are typically around a factor of 1.5 to 5 less than PELs for most hazardous substances; thus, of all the choices provided, 30 ug/meter^3 is the only tangible candidate. If an employee is exposed to lead for more than 8 hours in any work day, the PEL as a time-weighted average (TWA) for that day shall be reduced per the following formula:

PEL = (400) ÷ (total hours worked in the subject day)

123. D: There are no specific requirements stating that tags must be red, magenta, or black in color, or metallically attached in at least one location via a connection device, or must either display the term "High-Energy Hazard" or "Electrical Hazard" on its face. Tags must, however, be normalized (standardized) according to shape and size. In addition, they must be strong enough and attached well enough to prevent any inadvertent detachment and must always identify the employee(s) who affixed them.

124. C: The American National Standards Institute (ANSI) is the agency endowed with the ongoing responsibility of regularly setting standards for protective eyewear, including safety glasses, safety goggles, and other eye-related personal protective equipment (PPE).

125. A: If an employee death occurs as the result of a willful violation, as deemed by the courts, a fine of up to $250,000 can be imposed upon the guilty party or entity.

126. B: The constant for gravitational acceleration, in SI units, is 9.8 meters/second^2. In English-unit terms, this equates to 32.2 feet/second2. The constant depicts the acceleration on an object caused by the force of gravity. Neglecting potential frictional influences such as air resistance, all small bodies accelerate in a gravitational field at the same rate relative to their center of mass. This holds true regardless of the masses or compositions of the bodies.

127. A: Conditions adverse to quality are usually considered the most serious of all audit-finding classifications. Other types of findings from audits that fall into categories of lesser severity include: conditions not adverse to quality, observations, and opportunities for improvement. All categories would normally be entered, addressed, and closed out via the use of a robust corrective action program database.

128. C: Lost-time (i.e., DART) evaluations, incident trend assessments, and "lessons-learned" submittals are not considered safety interventions because they do not (probabilistically) have a direct effect on reducing the likelihood of an accident or event, although they may all potentially have an indirect effect to one extent or another. Measures such as installing design or engineering upgrades, enhancing safety program participation, and conducting robust training programs can all have a measurable, direct effect on lowering workplace incident risks.

129. C: Per OSHA 29 CFR 1910 Subpart D (Walking-Working Surfaces), a hole is defined as a gap or open space in a floor, roof, horizontal walking-working surface, or similar surface that is at least 2 inches (5 cm) in its least dimension.

130. B: Per ANSI/ASSE A1264.2, a coefficient of friction around 0.5 is considered moderately slippery. A value close to zero means that a surface is regarded as extremely slippery, while a value close to one is regarded as not slippery at all.

131. B: Rubber-insulated gloves used in electrical operations and construction work of more than 50 volts must meet subject requirements prescribed in ASTM D 120-09 (Standard Specification for Rubber Insulating Gloves) and must accordingly be categorized as Type-I.

132. D: OSHA requires that fall-protection equipment be used whenever a construction worker is at least 6 feet above the ground or if an employee is performing tasks while on a scaffold that is at least 10 feet above the ground.

133. C: Shelter-in-place procedures should include guidance on how to shut down ventilation systems and elevators, how to temporarily close off all exits and entrances, where building occupants should gather, and how to inform said occupants that an emergency has occurred. It is pivotal to note that during a shelter-in-place event, the primary intent is not to evacuate a work area or building (although at a later point it may ultimately be deemed by emergency response personnel that an evacuation may be necessary).

134. A: A usual first step in the conduct of a job safety analysis is to allocate some time to directly observe workers performing their tasks and to subsequently develop specific lists of actions and processes associated with the subject tasks at hand.

135. C: The primary goal of OSHA's voluntary protection program (VPP) is to methodically improve a company's health and safety management system by developing a strong bond (or partnership) between the employer and workforce within the domain of health and safety. A company must apply to OSHA to be considered and admitted to the VPP program. OSHA awards VPP star and merit program statuses to outperforming and overachieving organizations.

136. D: Structural failure occurs when a structure (or segment thereof) fails. The primary types of mechanisms usually responsible for initiating such a failure include corrosion (oxidation), buckling, extreme temperatures (hot and/or cold), tension, compression, bearing, shearing, creep, fatigue, and instability.

137. B: High-pressure fluids are used in such devices as fire hoses, fuel-injection mechanisms, concrete cleaners, and paint sprayers. Associated hazards include injection injuries, pressurized gas-impact injuries, and line-whipping.

138. C: Installed ramps must be constructed with a slope of less than 11 degrees for handicapped access.

139. B: The range of a data set is the numerical difference between the highest and lowest values in the set. Thus, 58 – 2 = 56.

140. C: A leading indicator is typically defined as an objective measure or metric that is used to assess proactive actions implemented with the goal of improving organizational performance.

141. C: Worker compensation laws have several key objectives; these include motivating employers to develop procedures that prevent or reduce accidents, replacing lost worker income, saving workers the time-consuming challenges of litigation, preventing injured workers from having to solicit charities, providing rapid medical treatment for sustained injuries, providing workers with rehabilitation options that enable a more efficient return to work, and encouraging accident investigations to ultimately prevent similar events from reoccurring. It should be noted that the goal of finding fault (culpability) for accident incidents is not a primary objective of worker compensation laws.

142. D: When a near miss occurs, the most advisable response is to address it as if it were an actual injury event by accordingly completing a root-cause analysis and setting forth action plans to prevent potential recurrences.

143. B: Routinely scheduled inspections are a vital part of an effective occupational safety and health program. As such, the frequency of inspections must be aligned with the degree of risk imposed by a subject operation in conjunction with regulatory requirements. Inspections that are not carried out at regular intervals are likely indicative of an insufficient occupational safety and health program.

144. D: The variance of a statistical population set is defined as the mathematical square of the standard deviation of that population set.

145. C: There are three fundamental types of air-supply equipment used in the workplace for ensuring good-quality, breathable air during periods where respiratory protection is required. These are supplied-air respirators (such as hose masks, air-line modules, hoods, and air-supplied suits); self-contained respirators (i.e., portable SCBA tanks); and air-purifying respirators (such as full-face or half-face respirators).

146. C: The pivotal factors to keep in mind when assessing potential chemical hazards are:

(1) compounds and materials that are generally known to be hazardous may not be considered dangerous below certain threshold concentrations, and (2) compounds and materials that aren't normally hazardous on their own may become hazardous when combined with other substances or when utilized in certain fashions.

147. D: Personal protective equipment (PPE) serves and only serves as a barrier between a worker and a hazard, but it does not remove the hazard. PPE should never be considered as a means for removing a hazard or for altogether perceiving a hazardous environment as a safe environment.

148. A: An electrical-based fire may be energized; therefore, it is critical not to douse it with any material that is capable of efficiently conducting electricity (i.e., water, foam, or metallic-based agents). Hence, carbon dioxide (as well as other suppressants such as FM-200 and dry-chemical powders) should be the first choice for extinguishing an electrical-based fire.

149. A: A repetitive strain injury (RSI) often results from long-term, cumulative trauma or stress to tendons, ligaments, nerves, joints, and/or muscles. Hands, arms, shoulders, and necks are usually the most affected areas to such injuries. Typical conditions associated with RSIs include epicondylitis, carpal-tunnel syndrome, trigger finger, bursitis, tendinitis, and fibromyalgia.

150. D: Infrared rays, microwaves, and radar waves are not forms of ionizing radiation; that is, they may excite electrons but do not have enough energy to ultimately strip or dislocate them from their respective shells (hence, creating the process of ionization). Forms of ionizing radiation include beta particles, alpha particles, gamma rays, X-rays, and neutrons. Ionizing radiation is the most hazardous type of radiation because it can chemically change particles, which can ultimately manifest in mutations and cancer.

151. A: Potential tripping hazards around a worksite can be substantially reduced in a number of ways. Such examples include avoiding altogether one- and two-step elevation changes, ensuring that flooring-transition areas are flush and level, robustly taping down or affixing electrical cords (or other media) if they cross over walkways, implementing robust housekeeping practices, and posting signs or warnings where there are known floor elevation changes, damaged materials, or temporary obstructions.

152. D: To effectively follow up on and correct audit findings, subject items should be grouped, as appropriate, into the following categories: (1) conditions adverse to quality (i.e., nonconformances); (2) areas of concern (i.e., potential high-risk items); and (3) opportunities for improvement.

153. C: A well-stocked first-aid-kit should include the following items: at least two sterile eye dressings, scissors, tweezers, rubbing alcohol, disposable sterile gloves, sterile gauze dressings, triangular bandages, mouthpieces, rolled bandages, cleansing wipes, sticky tape, safety pins, antihistamine tablets, distilled water, antiseptic cream, and an eye wash or bath.

154. B: Primary functions of machine guards are to keep body parts, clothing, and hair from coming into direct contact with hazardous machine parts (especially pinch points) as well as to prevent flying debris from striking workers. Secondary functions of guards include capturing dust, muffling machine noise, and containing machine-exhaust contaminants.

155. D: The domain of probabilistic risk assessment defines risk as the mathematical product of probability (i.e., frequency) and consequence. For example, if an accident has an annual probability of occurrence equal to 0.0001/year and the associated expected consequence is two fatalities resulting from that occurrence, then the annualized risk for such an occurrence is expected to be 0.0002 fatalities/year.

156. C: For a standard (normal) distribution of data, 68% of values will fall within ±1 standard deviation of the mean, 95% of values will fall within ±2 standard deviations of the mean, and 99.7% of values will fall within ±3 standard deviations of the mean. Such a distribution is typically known as a bell curve because its symmetrical shape resembles that of a bell.

157. A: An acute exposure refers to only a singular exposure (typically of high quantity or concentration) to a hazard, whereas a chronic exposure conventionally refers to repeated contact or interaction with a hazard (and can be at a variety of levels). Significant health effects can ultimately result from either type of exposure.

158. B: An asphyxiant is defined as a gas that displaces oxygen (in normally breathable air), thus potentially hindering the normal respiration cycle and ultimately decreasing the concentration of oxygen in the bloodstream. Carbon dioxide, nitrogen, helium, and argon are primary examples of asphyxiant gases.

159. D: Hazardous exposures in large-enough concentrations or frequencies can result in systemic effects to the body. Such effects may adversely impact body organs, functions, and systems—often severely.

160. D: There are three degrees of burns to which the human body is susceptible: first, second, and third. A first-degree burn is usually outer-layer superficial with some reddening and pain, with healing usually occurring within a week's time; a second-degree burn is deeper, characterized by blisters and pain, with healing usually occurring within a month's time; and a third-degree burn is usually depicted by all impacted skin layers being virtually destroyed, with healing potentially taking up to several months. Due to the potential destruction of nerve endings in the skin from a third-degree burn, it is often significantly less painful compared to a second-degree burn (and sometimes virtually pain-free [after the fact] depending upon the extent of nerve damage).

161. B: The most common types of workplace injuries are sprains and strains. Other common workplace injuries, however, include cuts, bruises, and bone fractures. Most such injuries usually occur due to slips, trips, falls, impacts, and overexertion.

162. A: In the workplace, the lower back (dorsal region) is the most frequently injured part of the body (primarily due to poor lifting techniques). After the back, the fingers, arms, ankles, and knees are usually the most commonly injured parts of the body.

163. B: Being struck by an object (blunt trauma) is unfortunately an all too common event within the workplace that can often result in serious injury or even death. An overexposure to hazardous materials (i.e., chemicals or radiation) is not overly common in the workplace, primarily due to the use of administrative or engineering controls, personal protective equipment (PPE), safety program protocols, and adherence to regulatory requirements. In a similar vein, due to the high-quality standards and reliability of today's PPE in most industries, associated failures rarely occur.

164. B: A lanyard's primary role within a fall-protection system is to connect a safety harness to an anchoring point. Lanyards absorb fall energy, so they reduce the impact load on a person when a fall is ultimately arrested.

165. C: On average, statistics regularly show that approximately 8% of workplace mishaps resulting in lost time are related to hand tool injuries.

166. C: There are three separate classifications or categories for flammable liquids: IA, IB, and IC. Propylene oxide is a Class IA flammable liquid (i.e., liquids that have flash points below 73°F [22.8°C] and boiling points below 100°F [37.8°C]). In contrast, Class IB flammable liquids are defined as those that have flash points below 73°F (22.8°C) and boiling points at or above 100°F (37.8°C), and Class IC liquids have flash points at or above 73°F (22.8°C) and boiling points below 100°F (37.8°C).

167. A: For work conducted in areas with high hazardous particulate concentrations (e.g., beryllium, silica, or lead), full-face (and often half-face) respirators are an appropriate choice for respiratory personal protective equipment (PPE). In addition to their high-efficiency air filtration capacity, full-face respirators also provide coverage to the eyes.

168. B: Per OSHA regulations, a respirator should be equipped with a blue-colored canister for providing protection against carbon monoxide gas.

169. A: A certified health physicist (CHP) is generally considered as a go-to subject matter expert regarding radiological hazards and doses in the workplace. A certified industrial hygienist (CIH), alternatively, would likely be the most qualified individual to assess a variety of hazards in the workplace and resultantly provide recommendations on how to effectively mitigate such hazards. A certified safety professional's (CSP's) breadth of expertise and training is typically commensurate with that of a CIH. A nuclear (professional) engineer's main area of focus is usually centered around innovating processes and systems that ultimately improve the quality, productivity, and safety of nuclear power plants.

170. C: The BCSP requirements for OHST recertification are the reporting of activities every 5 years and a minimum of 20 recertification points. Points may be accumulated through ongoing training, continuing education, memberships in safety organizations, work practices, publications, patents, and presentations.

171. D: Per OSHA 29 CFR 1926.56, general worksite (plant) areas and shops shall be illuminated at a light intensity level of 10 foot-candles or greater.

172. B: The term fit testing is used when specifically referring to respirator personal protective equipment (PPE). A fit test evaluates the quality of seal between the respirator's face piece and the user's face. It normally takes about 20 minutes to complete and should be performed on at least an annual basis. After passing a fit test, a worker must indefinitely use the exact same make, model, style, and size respirator on the job. A fit test should not be confused with a user seal check, which validates whether a respirator is properly seated to the face or needs to be readjusted each time the equipment is donned.

173. B: Welding, cutting, and brazing operations can entail many potential hazards, several of which may include potential eye damage from UV-light, burns, air contaminants from solder or other molten materials, and repetitive-strain injuries.

174. B: The security and privacy of worker personal health records are covered and protected under law per the Health Insurance Portability and Accountability Act's (HIPAA) Privacy Rule.

175. D: Lifting frequency for workers is normally calculated as the average number of lifts a worker performs over a 15-minute period.

176. C: A number of compressed-air (pneumatic) tools are regularly used in the workplace. Chippers, nail guns, saws, drills, sanders, diggers, and jackhammers comprise many of those that are most regularly utilized. Such tools often entail additional hazards that their non-pneumatic counterparts do not. Such examples include additional forces or inertia due to high air pressures, noise levels, pollutant emissions, shock potential, whipping-hose dangers, need for additional eye personal protective equipment (PPE), and chilled-air bursts.

177. A: Whenever an OSHA inspection occurs, the following items are deemed mandatory: (1) the employer must always be advised by the compliance officer as to the reason for the inspection; (2) the employer must accompany the compliance officer on the inspection; (3) the compliance officer must show official identification upon inspection; and (4) the employer must be assured by the compliance officer that any trade secrets observed during the inspection will remain confidential.

178. A: A severity rate (SR) of 36.90 is calculated for the scenario of five recordable injuries with one of these resulting in 40 days of lost time and a total number of workforce hours worked equal to 216,800.

$$SR = \text{(number of lost workdays x 200,000)} \div \text{(total number of hours worked)}$$
$$= (40 \times 200{,}000) \div (216{,}800)$$
$$= 36.90$$

179. C: A strong acid typically has a pH around 1, and a strong base typically has a pH around 14; in contrast, a weak acid usually has a pH in the range of 3 to 6.9 and a weak base usually has a pH in the range of 7.1 to 11. Strong acids and bases are very caustic and usually present numerous potential hazards to human health if exposure occurs via ingestion, inhalation, or externally; weak acids and bases on the hand, although still somewhat hazardous to these regards, are typically not nearly as dangerous as their "stronger" counterparts. Whether weak or strong, however, it should always be noted that many are chemically poisonous. Examples of weak acids include acetic and carbonic, whereas examples of weak bases include ammonia and phosphine.

180. A: There are numerous particulate agents or substances in the workplace to which workers may potentially be exposed that are tied to the manifestation of specific diseases and/or disorders if taken up. Such agents and substances include cadmium, which can lead to a host of serious systemic conditions; beryllium, which can lead to berylliosis; and silica, which can lead to silicosis. Other well-known toxic and hazardous materials to be aware of in the workplace include lead, mercury, and asbestos.

181. D: There are several potential violation categories which exist under OSHA, including a serious violation (a violation that entails a significant possibility that death or serious physical harm can result); a willful violation (a violation that an individual or employer intentionally and knowingly commits); a failure-to-abate violation (a failure to correct a prior condition); a repeated violation (a violation that is found to be very similar to a previous violation); and an other-than-serious violation (a violation that has a direct relationship to health and safety but in all probability would not cause death or serious injury).

182. D: The term TLV, in regard to hazardous chemical exposure, stands for threshold limit value. It is defined as the consensus level to which a worker can be exposed (to a given chemical) on a daily basis for a working lifetime, likely without the materialization of adverse health effects. TLV is a reserved term of the American Conference of Governmental Industrial Hygienists (ACGIH).

183. C: The US FDA is responsible for protecting the general public from potential hazards associated with the use of all pharmaceutical products as well as foodstuffs, cosmetics, organics, or any other products that are potentially used for remedial purposes.

184. C: The preponderance of laws that involve worker health and safety fall under the purview of civil law. The Occupational Safety and Health Act of 1970 is the chief civil law that is presently in use for protecting worker health and safety and is regularly enforced by OSHA. Thus, injured workers should normally seek counsel from civil attorneys if they are seeking compensation due to alleged harm incurred on the job that could have been avoided with an appropriate level of corporate engagement.

185. D: Federal safety-regulating agencies, such as OSHA and MSHA, normally track a variety of metrics related to worker injuries and illnesses. Such metrics typically include frequencies of work-related deaths, frequencies of major injuries, frequencies of job transfers, and frequencies of restricted duty.

186. B: The OSHA Classification System for Occupational Illnesses and Conditions includes several categories, including radiation-related disorders or conditions, respiratory-related disorders or conditions, epidermal-related disorders or conditions, toxicity-related disorders or conditions, and repetitive-motion/ergonomic-related disorders or conditions (e.g., RSIs).

187. A: Per NAAQS protocol (40 CFR 50), the maximum allowable criteria pollutant concentration for lead (Pb) is 0.15 μg/meter^3 over a 3-month period.

188. C: The US Bureau of Labor Statistics is responsible for distributing statistical information pertaining to job-related injuries and illnesses. Other agencies, however, such as the US Occupational Safety and Health Administration and the US National Institute of Occupational Safety and Health often cite such published statistics in support of their enforcement initiatives, missions, campaigns, and outreach programs.

189. B: There are several characteristic shapes of frequency curves that exist in the realm of graphical statistics. These include (left or right) skewed, j shaped, multimodal, U shaped, and symmetrical (such as with a Gaussian normal distribution).

190. A: Injury information resulting from an incident should be reported by corporate health and safety management personnel as soon as possible after an occurrence. Specific OSHA protocol (per 29 CFR 1904.39) requires, however, that any work-related deaths must be reported within an 8-hour window. Any work-related amputations (including fingers or toes), loss(es) of an eye, or inpatient hospitalizations must be reported within 24 hours of an incident.

191. D: Conditions adverse to quality are usually considered, by far, the most serious of all audit-finding classifications. Other types of audit findings that fall into categories of respectively lesser severity include the following (in order): conditions not adverse to quality, observations, and opportunities for improvement. All categories would normally be entered, addressed, and closed out via the use of an independent corrective-action program database.

192. C: In the following Cartesian data-point set: [(−0.4, −1.2), (2, 5.7), (4, 11.8), (7, 20), (9, 28.1), (12, 29), (15, 46.1), and (19, 56)], the point (12, 29) would be considered an anomaly compared to all of the others. This can be demonstrated by plotting all of the subject values via a scatter plot and noting that all of the other points essentially construct a straight line. The point (12, 29), however, falls well outside of this line, thereby denoting it as an anomaly with respect to the rest of the data set.

193. C: Techniques such as case study deployment, peer collaboration, and role-play are commonly implemented when attempting to effectively train supervisors and upper management on protocols that are not specifically laid out in procedural guidance or other criteria.

194. A: Commonly utilized conflict resolution methods typically employed in industry include adjudicative resolution, consensual dispute resolution, and legislative resolution. These methods can discretionarily invoke the use of arbitrators, negotiators, and possibly even the court system, as deemed applicable.

195. D: Calculations and analyses performed by insurance companies that assess company loss-rate records for establishing worker compensation premiums are conventionally known as experience modifiers.

196. A: The office warden is usually responsible for taking roll calls during a shelter in place or a building evacuation. Such roll calls help ensure that all employees are accounted for (i.e., present or not present) during a potential emergency situation.

197. B: According to Herzberg's theory of behavior, a worker's desired extrinsic outcomes typically include the following tenets: job-security, monetary income, and safe and comfortable working conditions.

198. D: Hepatitis-C contracted in the workplace from an inadvertent needle-stick accident would be categorized as a privacy case on an OSHA 300 form, whereby the employee's name is not recorded on the form. Other scenarios that could qualify as privacy cases include injury to the reproductive organs, a mental illness or condition, an injury or illness resulting from a sexual assault, HIV-infection, or tuberculosis.

199. A: According to Maslow's hierarchy of needs, personal facets such as morality, problem solving, creativity, spontaneity, and lack of prejudice all fall under the human need of self-actualization.

200. D: A directive-autocrat leadership personality does not typically provide employees the opportunity to contribute to decision-making processes and usually affords subordinates a minimal degree of latitude in carrying out their tasks (i.e., the micromanager). Other types of leadership personalities include permissive-autocrat (semi-liberal style), directive-democrat (semi-liberal style), and permissive-democrat (liberal, flexible, and open style).

How to Overcome Test Anxiety

Just the thought of taking a test is enough to make most people a little nervous. A test is an important event that can have a long-term impact on your future, so it's important to take it seriously and it's natural to feel anxious about performing well. But just because anxiety is normal, that doesn't mean that it's helpful in test taking, or that you should simply accept it as part of your life. Anxiety can have a variety of effects. These effects can be mild, like making you feel slightly nervous, or severe, like blocking your ability to focus or remember even a simple detail.

If you experience test anxiety—whether severe or mild—it's important to know how to beat it. To discover this, first you need to understand what causes test anxiety.

Causes of Test Anxiety

While we often think of anxiety as an uncontrollable emotional state, it can actually be caused by simple, practical things. One of the most common causes of test anxiety is that a person does not feel adequately prepared for their test. This feeling can be the result of many different issues such as poor study habits or lack of organization, but the most common culprit is time management. Starting to study too late, failing to organize your study time to cover all of the material, or being distracted while you study will mean that you're not well prepared for the test. This may lead to cramming the night before, which will cause you to be physically and mentally exhausted for the test. Poor time management also contributes to feelings of stress, fear, and hopelessness as you realize you are not well prepared but don't know what to do about it.

Other times, test anxiety is not related to your preparation for the test but comes from unresolved fear. This may be a past failure on a test, or poor performance on tests in general. It may come from comparing yourself to others who seem to be performing better or from the stress of living up to expectations. Anxiety may be driven by fears of the future—how failure on this test would affect your educational and career goals. These fears are often completely irrational, but they can still negatively impact your test performance.

Elements of Test Anxiety

As mentioned earlier, test anxiety is considered to be an emotional state, but it has physical and mental components as well. Sometimes you may not even realize that you are suffering from test anxiety until you notice the physical symptoms. These can include trembling hands, rapid heartbeat, sweating, nausea, and tense muscles. Extreme anxiety may lead to fainting or vomiting. Obviously, any of these symptoms can have a negative impact on testing. It is important to recognize them as soon as they begin to occur so that you can address the problem before it damages your performance.

The mental components of test anxiety include trouble focusing and inability to remember learned information. During a test, your mind is on high alert, which can help you recall information and stay focused for an extended period of time. However, anxiety interferes with your mind's natural processes, causing you to blank out, even on the questions you know well. The strain of testing during anxiety makes it difficult to stay focused, especially on a test that may take several hours. Extreme anxiety can take a huge mental toll, making it difficult not only to recall test information but even to understand the test questions or pull your thoughts together.

Effects of Test Anxiety

Test anxiety is like a disease—if left untreated, it will get progressively worse. Anxiety leads to poor performance, and this reinforces the feelings of fear and failure, which in turn lead to poor performances on subsequent tests. It can grow from a mild nervousness to a crippling condition. If allowed to progress, test anxiety can have a big impact on your schooling, and consequently on your future.

Test anxiety can spread to other parts of your life. Anxiety on tests can become anxiety in any stressful situation, and blanking on a test can turn into panicking in a job situation. But fortunately, you don't have to let anxiety rule your testing and determine your grades. There are a number of relatively simple steps you can take to move past anxiety and function normally on a test and in the rest of life.

Physical Steps for Beating Test Anxiety

While test anxiety is a serious problem, the good news is that it can be overcome. It doesn't have to control your ability to think and remember information. While it may take time, you can begin taking steps today to beat anxiety.

Just as your first hint that you may be struggling with anxiety comes from the physical symptoms, the first step to treating it is also physical. Rest is crucial for having a clear, strong mind. If you are tired, it is much easier to give in to anxiety. But if you establish good sleep habits, your body and mind will be ready to perform optimally, without the strain of exhaustion. Additionally, sleeping well helps you to retain information better, so you're more likely to recall the answers when you see the test questions.

Getting good sleep means more than going to bed on time. It's important to allow your brain time to relax. Take study breaks from time to time so it doesn't get overworked, and don't study right before bed. Take time to rest your mind before trying to rest your body, or you may find it difficult to fall asleep.

Along with sleep, other aspects of physical health are important in preparing for a test. Good nutrition is vital for good brain function. Sugary foods and drinks may give a burst of energy but this burst is followed by a crash, both physically and emotionally. Instead, fuel your body with protein and vitamin-rich foods.

Also, drink plenty of water. Dehydration can lead to headaches and exhaustion, especially if your brain is already under stress from the rigors of the test. Particularly if your test is a long one, drink water during the breaks. And if possible, take an energy-boosting snack to eat between sections.

Along with sleep and diet, a third important part of physical health is exercise. Maintaining a steady workout schedule is helpful, but even taking 5-minute study breaks to walk can help get your blood pumping faster and clear your head. Exercise also releases endorphins, which contribute to a positive feeling and can help combat test anxiety.

When you nurture your physical health, you are also contributing to your mental health. If your body is healthy, your mind is much more likely to be healthy as well. So take time to rest, nourish your body with healthy food and water, and get moving as much as possible. Taking these physical steps will make you stronger and more able to take the mental steps necessary to overcome test anxiety.

Mental Steps for Beating Test Anxiety

Working on the mental side of test anxiety can be more challenging, but as with the physical side, there are clear steps you can take to overcome it. As mentioned earlier, test anxiety often stems from lack of preparation, so the obvious solution is to prepare for the test. Effective studying may be the most important weapon you have for beating test anxiety, but you can and should employ several other mental tools to combat fear.

First, boost your confidence by reminding yourself of past success—tests or projects that you aced. If you're putting as much effort into preparing for this test as you did for those, there's no reason you should expect to fail here. Work hard to prepare; then trust your preparation.

Second, surround yourself with encouraging people. It can be helpful to find a study group, but be sure that the people you're around will encourage a positive attitude. If you spend time with others who are anxious or cynical, this will only contribute to your own anxiety. Look for others who are motivated to study hard from a desire to succeed, not from a fear of failure.

Third, reward yourself. A test is physically and mentally tiring, even without anxiety, and it can be helpful to have something to look forward to. Plan an activity following the test, regardless of the outcome, such as going to a movie or getting ice cream.

When you are taking the test, if you find yourself beginning to feel anxious, remind yourself that you know the material. Visualize successfully completing the test. Then take a few deep, relaxing breaths and return to it. Work through the questions carefully but with confidence, knowing that you are capable of succeeding.

Developing a healthy mental approach to test taking will also aid in other areas of life. Test anxiety affects more than just the actual test—it can be damaging to your mental health and even contribute to depression. It's important to beat test anxiety before it becomes a problem for more than testing.

Study Strategy

Being prepared for the test is necessary to combat anxiety, but what does being prepared look like? You may study for hours on end and still not feel prepared. What you need is a strategy for test prep. The next few pages outline our recommended steps to help you plan out and conquer the challenge of preparation.

STEP 1: SCOPE OUT THE TEST

Learn everything you can about the format (multiple choice, essay, etc.) and what will be on the test. Gather any study materials, course outlines, or sample exams that may be available. Not only will this help you to prepare, but knowing what to expect can help to alleviate test anxiety.

STEP 2: MAP OUT THE MATERIAL

Look through the textbook or study guide and make note of how many chapters or sections it has. Then divide these over the time you have. For example, if a book has 15 chapters and you have five days to study, you need to cover three chapters each day. Even better, if you have the time, leave an extra day at the end for overall review after you have gone through the material in depth.

If time is limited, you may need to prioritize the material. Look through it and make note of which sections you think you already have a good grasp on, and which need review. While you are studying, skim quickly through the familiar sections and take more time on the challenging parts.

Write out your plan so you don't get lost as you go. Having a written plan also helps you feel more in control of the study, so anxiety is less likely to arise from feeling overwhelmed at the amount to cover.

STEP 3: GATHER YOUR TOOLS

Decide what study method works best for you. Do you prefer to highlight in the book as you study and then go back over the highlighted portions? Or do you type out notes of the important information? Or is it helpful to make flashcards that you can carry with you? Assemble the pens, index cards, highlighters, post-it notes, and any other materials you may need so you won't be distracted by getting up to find things while you study.

If you're having a hard time retaining the information or organizing your notes, experiment with different methods. For example, try color-coding by subject with colored pens, highlighters, or post-it notes. If you learn better by hearing, try recording yourself reading your notes so you can listen while in the car, working out, or simply sitting at your desk. Ask a friend to quiz you from your flashcards, or try teaching someone the material to solidify it in your mind.

STEP 4: CREATE YOUR ENVIRONMENT

It's important to avoid distractions while you study. This includes both the obvious distractions like visitors and the subtle distractions like an uncomfortable chair (or a too-comfortable couch that makes you want to fall asleep). Set up the best study environment possible: good lighting and a comfortable work area. If background music helps you focus, you may want to turn it on, but otherwise keep the room quiet. If you are using a computer to take notes, be sure you don't have any other windows open, especially applications like social media, games, or anything else that could distract you. Silence your phone and turn off notifications. Be sure to keep water close by so you stay hydrated while you study (but avoid unhealthy drinks and snacks).

Also, take into account the best time of day to study. Are you freshest first thing in the morning? Try to set aside some time then to work through the material. Is your mind clearer in the afternoon or evening? Schedule your study session then. Another method is to study at the same time of day that you will take the test, so that your brain gets used to working on the material at that time and will be ready to focus at test time.

STEP 5: STUDY!

Once you have done all the study preparation, it's time to settle into the actual studying. Sit down, take a few moments to settle your mind so you can focus, and begin to follow your study plan. Don't give in to distractions or let yourself procrastinate. This is your time to prepare so you'll be ready to fearlessly approach the test. Make the most of the time and stay focused.

Of course, you don't want to burn out. If you study too long you may find that you're not retaining the information very well. Take regular study breaks. For example, taking five minutes out of every hour to walk briskly, breathing deeply and swinging your arms, can help your mind stay fresh.

As you get to the end of each chapter or section, it's a good idea to do a quick review. Remind yourself of what you learned and work on any difficult parts. When you feel that you've mastered the material, move on to the next part. At the end of your study session, briefly skim through your notes again.

But while review is helpful, cramming last minute is NOT. If at all possible, work ahead so that you won't need to fit all your study into the last day. Cramming overloads your brain with more information than it can process and retain, and your tired mind may struggle to recall even previously learned information when it is overwhelmed with last-minute study. Also, the urgent nature of cramming and the stress placed on your brain contribute to anxiety. You'll be more likely to go to the test feeling unprepared and having trouble thinking clearly.

So don't cram, and don't stay up late before the test, even just to review your notes at a leisurely pace. Your brain needs rest more than it needs to go over the information again. In fact, plan to finish your studies by noon or early afternoon the day before the test. Give your brain the rest of the day to relax or focus on other things, and get a good night's sleep. Then you will be fresh for the test and better able to recall what you've studied.

STEP 6: TAKE A PRACTICE TEST

Many courses offer sample tests, either online or in the study materials. This is an excellent resource to check whether you have mastered the material, as well as to prepare for the test format and environment.

Check the test format ahead of time: the number of questions, the type (multiple choice, free response, etc.), and the time limit. Then create a plan for working through them. For example, if you have 30 minutes to take a 60-question test, your limit is 30 seconds per question. Spend less time on the questions you know well so that you can take more time on the difficult ones.

If you have time to take several practice tests, take the first one open book, with no time limit. Work through the questions at your own pace and make sure you fully understand them. Gradually work up to taking a test under test conditions: sit at a desk with all study materials put away and set a timer. Pace yourself to make sure you finish the test with time to spare and go back to check your answers if you have time.

After each test, check your answers. On the questions you missed, be sure you understand why you missed them. Did you misread the question (tests can use tricky wording)? Did you forget the information? Or was it something you hadn't learned? Go back and study any shaky areas that the practice tests reveal.

Taking these tests not only helps with your grade, but also aids in combating test anxiety. If you're already used to the test conditions, you're less likely to worry about it, and working through tests until you're scoring well gives you a confidence boost. Go through the practice tests until you feel comfortable, and then you can go into the test knowing that you're ready for it.

Test Tips

On test day, you should be confident, knowing that you've prepared well and are ready to answer the questions. But aside from preparation, there are several test day strategies you can employ to maximize your performance.

First, as stated before, get a good night's sleep the night before the test (and for several nights before that, if possible). Go into the test with a fresh, alert mind rather than staying up late to study.

Try not to change too much about your normal routine on the day of the test. It's important to eat a nutritious breakfast, but if you normally don't eat breakfast at all, consider eating just a protein bar. If you're a coffee drinker, go ahead and have your normal coffee. Just make sure you time it so that the caffeine doesn't wear off right in the middle of your test. Avoid sugary beverages, and drink enough water to stay hydrated but not so much that you need a restroom break 10 minutes into the test. If your test isn't first thing in the morning, consider going for a walk or doing a light workout before the test to get your blood flowing.

Allow yourself enough time to get ready, and leave for the test with plenty of time to spare so you won't have the anxiety of scrambling to arrive in time. Another reason to be early is to select a good seat. It's helpful to sit away from doors and windows, which can be distracting. Find a good seat, get out your supplies, and settle your mind before the test begins.

When the test begins, start by going over the instructions carefully, even if you already know what to expect. Make sure you avoid any careless mistakes by following the directions.

Then begin working through the questions, pacing yourself as you've practiced. If you're not sure on an answer, don't spend too much time on it, and don't let it shake your confidence. Either skip it and come back later, or eliminate as many wrong answers as possible and guess among the remaining ones. Don't dwell on these questions as you continue—put them out of your mind and focus on what lies ahead.

Be sure to read all of the answer choices, even if you're sure the first one is the right answer. Sometimes you'll find a better one if you keep reading. But don't second-guess yourself if you do immediately know the answer. Your gut instinct is usually right. Don't let test anxiety rob you of the information you know.

If you have time at the end of the test (and if the test format allows), go back and review your answers. Be cautious about changing any, since your first instinct tends to be correct, but make sure you didn't misread any of the questions or accidentally mark the wrong answer choice. Look over any you skipped and make an educated guess.

At the end, leave the test feeling confident. You've done your best, so don't waste time worrying about your performance or wishing you could change anything. Instead, celebrate the successful completion of this test. And finally, use this test to learn how to deal with anxiety even better next time.

Review Video: Test Anxiety Visit mometrix.com/academy and enter code: 100340

Important Qualification

Not all anxiety is created equal. If your test anxiety is causing major issues in your life beyond the classroom or testing center, or if you are experiencing troubling physical symptoms related to your anxiety, it may be a sign of a serious physiological or psychological condition. If this sounds like your situation, we strongly encourage you to seek professional help.

Online Resources

Due to our efforts to try to keep this book to a manageable length, we've created a link that will give you access to all of your online resources:

mometrix.com/resources719/ohst

It's Your Moment, Let's Celebrate It!

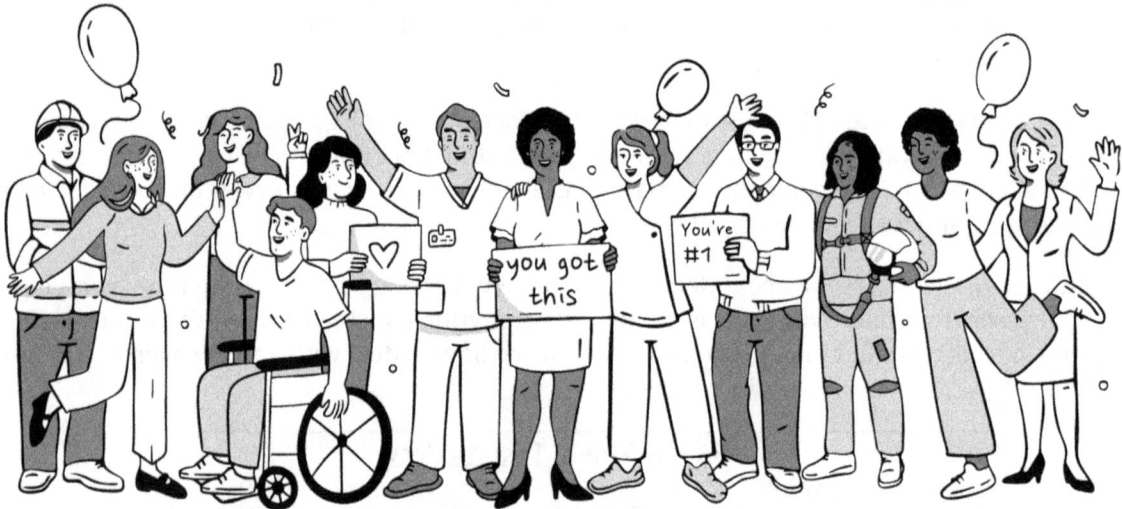

Share your story @mometrixtestpreparation